Academic Medicine:
A Guide for Clinicians

D0830303

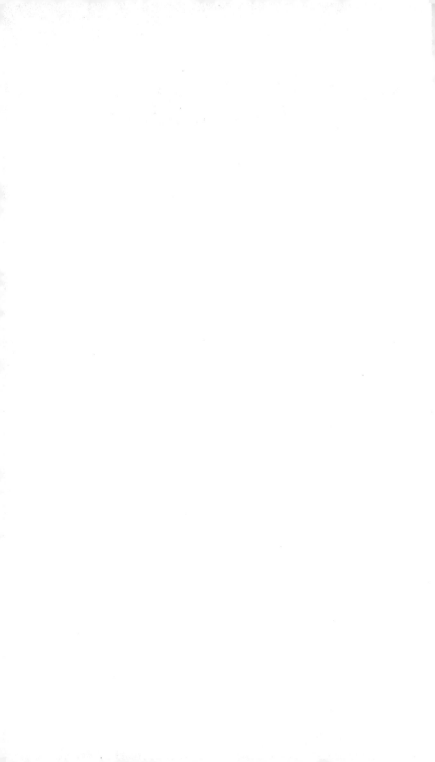

Academic Medicine:
A Guide for Clinicians

Robert B. Taylor, MD

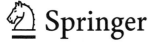 Springer

Robert B. Taylor, MD
Department of Family Medicine
Oregon Health & Science University School of Medicine
Portland, Oregon 97239-3098
USA
taylorr@ohsu.edu

W
19
T245a
2006

Library of Congress Control Number: 2005932558

ISBN-10: 0-387-28956-9
ISBN-13: 978-0387-28956-4

Printed on acid-free paper.

Printed in the United States of America.   (MP/BP)

9 8 7 6 5 4 3 2 1

springer.com

If you want to know what lies ahead on the trail, ask
someone who has made the journey and returned.
Old Chinese proverb

My advice is to be true to yourself, pursue your dream, and
keep your options open. This advice is for anyone in
medicine—whether you are a medical student or an
attending-level clinician. It is never too late to make the
choice to be happier in life.
Advice from one of the book's contributors

The improbability of the events depicted in this [book] is
the surest indication that they actually did occur.
Modified from the declaration at the start of the HBO movie
And Starring Pancho Villa as Himself.
The story tells how the Mexican revolutionary collaborated
with a U.S. film company to spread his message.
I will return to this quotation in the last chapter of the book.

Preface

What makes a successful academic clinician?
Good judgment.

How do you get good judgment?
Experience.

How do you get experience?
Making mistakes.

Is making mistakes really the best way to learn?

There are three important life decisions when mistakes could be especially costly for the clinician: Whom (or if) you marry, your specialty choice, and the path of your career. I really can't help you with the first decision, and your specialty choice has probably already been made. This book is about the third decision—the direction of your career path. If you decide to become a faculty member at an academic medical center, your career trajectory will depend on the choices you make (or don't make) when you encounter the diverse opportunities that arise throughout your professional life. I hope to help you make good decisions and avoid the common mistakes.

This book is intended to be a newcomer's guide to the academic medical center and the teaching hospital. It is written from the viewpoint of those who have walked the trail and learned from experience. As one very new faculty member remarked when I told him about plans for the book, "It would have been great to have this information last year, when I was looking at faculty positions. When you are finishing your residency or fellowship, you don't know what you don't know."

The book contains specific tactical advice for readers in each stage of considering or beginning an academic medicine career. Readers who would benefit from this book include medical students, residents and fellows considering academic careers, and junior faculty members in all specialties. In fact, I have found some of the latter group, junior faculty members, to be surprisingly uninformed about the environment in which they work, perhaps because they think themselves too busy to have time to learn about faculty development, scholarship, and promotion. Practicing physicians considering a move to academic practice and teaching should read this book before mailing a curriculum vitae. The chief qualifications for readership are that you actually see patients and that you are considering or beginning a teaching career; that is, becoming or being an *academic clinician*.

This book is the view from 7500 feet. Bob Bomengen, MD, is a physician friend who left private practice to spend a year in our clinical department at the Oregon Health & Science University. Bob's practice is in Lakeview, Oregon, a frontier community of about 3000 persons. His hobby is flying his single-engine Cessna and, from his small plane, he can see the towns, streets, individual houses, and people. He can see rivers and trees, cattle and horses. He can see things you can't see in a huge jet at 35,000 feet, from which the view is likely to be a cloudy blur. Academic medical center chief executive officers, university presidents, and deans live at 35,000 feet. Clinicians like Dr. Bob Bomengen and those who make the move after residency or fellowship enter academic medicine at a much lower altitude. This book is written for these individuals—those pondering or starting an academic career and wanting to learn about the world of clinicians who also teach and sometimes do research and write scholarly articles and books.

This book will be especially useful for academic clinicians in their first 5 years on faculty. These, generally younger, academicians can also see the trees and rivers but still seem to bump into limbs and get their feet damp, sometimes in hot water. Residency and fellowship training does not adequately prepare the trainee for an academic role. The change from learner to faculty member is profound, and this book can help prevent early career missteps.

This is the book I wish had been available when I entered academic medicine in 1978, not knowing the meaning of the acronym NOGA or the difference between hard and soft money. Later in the book, I'll tell you why and how I began an academic career that led me to two of America's premier academic medical centers, and I will share some personal adventures over the past 27 years. The book also describes the experiences of others, as well as offering practical advice as to how you can improve key skills in teaching, scholarship, grant-getting, administration, and, yes, clinical abilities.

A key feature of this book is the inclusion of responses to a questionnaire sent to academic clinicians in various specialties and geographic locations. Questions included: "What attracted you to an academic medical career?" "What has been the surprise about your work in an academic medical center?" And "What is some advice you would give the clinician entering academics?" Contributors' stories set the stage for concepts presented in the book. The contributors have my profound thanks for telling about their lives.

The book also includes comments and opinions from scores of other academicians. Instead of answering formal, structured questions, these clinicians provided brief comments, short anecdotes, and lessons learned from experience. I am grateful for what they have brought to this project.

I want also to thank two special people. One is Coelleda O'Neil, who helped with the figures and tables in the book. The other is my wife and colleague, Anita D. Taylor, MA Ed, an experienced author in her own right who consulted liberally in all phases of writing and did not hesitate to tell me when sentences and paragraphs "needed some more work."

I hope that there will be a second edition of this book some day. Based on that possibility, I invite you to share your thoughts, experiences, perhaps even a mistake—in short, your adventures in academic medicine.

Robert B. Taylor, MD
Portland, Oregon

Contents

Contributors

The contributors to this book represent a "convenience sample" of physicians with academic experience. The list was not randomly selected, and I am sure there is some selection bias. I did, however, obtain diversity in regard to geography, specialty, academic setting, gender, age, and rank.

The contributors listed below represent:

- Two countries: United States and Canada
- Eight states in the United States and one Canadian province
- Eleven medical specialties and subspecialties
- Ten academic medical centers
- Faculty ranks ranging from instructor to tenured professor

The ages of contributors vary from 31 years to 72 years, and the faculty ranks range from instructor to professor. There are an assistant dean, two associate deans, and a former dean. One contributor is on the threshold of an academic career, one is "easing out," and one has recently left the academic setting. Some contributors entered academic medicine right out of training; others came from private practice settings. I believe that each of these individuals represents an important perspective.

I thank the following contributors:

Elizabeth C. Clark, MD, MPH
Brian J. Cole, MD, MBA
Cliff Coleman, MD, MPH
John W. Ely, MD
Ray F. Friedman, MD
James D. MacLowry, MD
Amit Mehta, MD, FRCPc, DABR, DCBNC
Thomas E. Norris, MD

Molly Osborne, MD, PhD
Kevin Patrick, MD, MS
Paul M. Paulman, MD
Heather Paladine, MD
John Saultz, MD
Joseph E. Scherger, MD, MPH
Ronald Schneeweiss, MB, ChB
Elizabeth Steiner, MD
Harry S. Strothers III, MD, MMM
Christopher B. White, MD
Thad Wilkins, MD
Ronald B. Workman, Jr., MD

About This Book

We are about to embark on a journey. The book's contributors and I will be your guides as you, a clinician, enter the world of academia. The culture shock can be like my trip to the People's Republic of China in 1980, just as that country opened to foreigners after being "closed" for decades. The Chinese people I encountered at that time lived very differently than me; they dressed differently, spoke a language that I could not understand, and had a value system that was much unlike mine. But I was a tourist; I was not planning to live there. I could observe the people and the culture, but I didn't attempt to become one of them.

The resident, fellow, or clinician in private practice who becomes an academician soon finds some things that are different. During your first few years on faculty, you become aware of academia's idiosyncrasies. The language can be new and confusing—a whole new set of jargon, abbreviations, and acronyms. Examples include effort allocation, formative feedback, indirect costs, RFP, NOGA, and XYZ. But what is really different is the value system. In academia, the *summum bonum* is the creation of new knowledge. Grant-getting skills may be seen as more important than teaching abilities. Clinical expertise, although important, is not always at the top of the values pyramid.

At this point, let us agree on some definitions: A *teaching hospital* is a setting for patient care that also has one or more educational programs. According to the *Journal of the American Medical Association*, teaching hospitals are "hospitals that are affiliated with medical schools and serve as 'classrooms' for physician, nurses, and other health care workers in training."[1] A *medical school* has faculty members that teach medical students; there may also be some related training programs, such as physicians' assistants. An *academic medical center* (AMC) includes a medical school that trains physicians, a system for delivering health care services, and research activities involving laboratory science, clinical investigation, or both.[2] At an AMC, you will probably find various specialized clinics, research centers, master's and PhD degree programs, and more. For example, I work at the Oregon Health & Science University (OHSU), which has schools of medicine, nursing, and dentistry, plus five hospitals and educational programs in a variety of health-related areas.

Each AMC is unique in various ways. You will see this fact illustrated throughout the book. Variations include the organizational structure, faculty compensation system, clinical practice plan, promotion and tenure guidelines, the unwritten rules, and even the culture. A favorite aphorism is, If you have seen one academic medical center, you have seen one. For example, in a state university system, you may be a candidate for promotion to associate professor of medicine and find an English literature professor on the promotion and tenure committee that evaluates your fitness for advancement in rank. This is not the case at Oregon Health & Science University; my school of medicine is not part of the University of Oregon or Oregon State University and thus has no departments of English literature or ancient history, but we do have students working toward a variety of degrees, including PhD, master of public health, master of science, and master of nursing.

The book tells about life as an academic clinician, a term that I will explain further in Chapter 1. In the first four chapters, I will discuss the academic career decision, life in academia, and how to get the job you want. In Chapter 5, I will tell about basic skills needed—clinical practice, teaching, and scholarship. Chapter 6 presents some introductory guidance about more advanced academic skills; these include conducting research, assembling a grant proposal, and writing for publication. Administrative skills and academic medicine success skills are described in Chapters 7 and 8. Tables in these chapters show where to look to learn more. Chapter 9 gives advice on how to manage your career and your life. The stories of those who have walked the trail before you, and some lessons learned along the way, are found in Chapter 10. The Glossary explains the sometimes-arcane abbreviations and educational idioms encountered in academic medicine.

The experiential basis for the advice given is the collection of stories offered by the book's 20 contributors, whom I estimate have a combined total of more than 300 career years in academic medicine. The contributors represent 11 medical specialties and subspecialties in academic medical centers across North America. I used network research to assemble the panel, who range in academic experience from first-year junior faculty to seasoned full professors. In compiling their comments and anecdotes, I have tried to make the book as authoritative and yet as "personal" as I can.

In addition to sharing personal experiences, I have made liberal use of the medical literature, especially in regard to teaching, scholarship, research, grant getting, and other academic endeavors. Also, because I believe that all clinicians should have interests outside of medicine, in the coming pages we will visit the island of Cos and the Oregon Trail, *Tyrannosaurus rex* and St. John's wort, Mark Twain and Marcus Aurelius, and the alligator that ate my nephew's dog.

Just before we depart on our journey, I should tell you about your chief guide—me. I think this is important because you must always assess the source of any advice you receive. You should know the "expert's" background, experience, and, if possible, that person's biases and what the origins of those viewpoints might be.

So here goes: I am a family physician and have been a clinician for 43 years. After my training and required uniformed service time, I was in group practice in the small town of New Paltz, New York, for 4 years, and then in rural solo practice in a nearby village for 10 years. In this clinical setting, I began writing and editing medical books. This scholarship is what prompted me to sell the office that I had built and move my family from the Hudson Valley of New York State to Winston-Salem, North Carolina, where I joined the faculty of the Bowman Gray School of Medicine of Wake Forest University. I believe that moving from private, solo practice to academics made me keenly aware of the cultural differences in the two settings. In the early years, I experienced some painful lessons as I struggled to fathom academic medicine's complexity, quirks, and unwritten rules of conduct.

I spent 6 years at Wake Forest University School of Medicine, learning the ropes of academic medicine, before deciding that I wanted to be a chairman of a medical school clinical department. And then, after interviewing at a number of medical schools around the country, in 1984 I became the second chairman of the Department of Family Medicine at the Oregon Health & Science University School of Medicine in Portland, Oregon. I held this position for 14 years, and then in 1998 I resigned the chairmanship and assumed my current position as professor emeritus. During my academic career, I have worked with seven medical school deans, which—do the math—speaks to the relatively short tenures of those who lead our medical faculties. Also, along the way I wrote and edited 23 medical reference books, held the position of chair of the Medical Board of the Medical Staff at our University Hospital, and served with the National Board of Medical Examiners and in leadership roles in several national and international organizations.

In addition to providing vital information to guide early career decisions, this book has a "hidden agenda," which I hereby share with you. This goal is to enhance the job satisfaction and status of the growing number of clinician-educators in academic medicine. I hope to do so by encouraging some scholarly activity in addition to clinical care and teaching, by showing them how to fit into the academic milieu, and by guiding these faculty members in strategies to succeed in an apparently benign, yet highly competitive, environment.

Now we're ready to start. Chapter 1 discusses the early steps in an academic career, beginning with a very important decision as to what we will call the clinician who teaches students and residents and may do some research, writing, or academic administration.

Enjoy the adventure.

REFERENCES

1. Stevens LM, Lynm C, Glass RM. Academic health centers. JAMA 2004;292:1134.
2. Aaron HJ. The plight of academic medical centers: Policy Brief #59. Washington, DC, The Brookings Institution, 2000.

1

Deciding on an Academic Career

> *Medicine is the oldest learned profession in the world and it is rooted in the past. Each successive generation of doctors stands, as it were, upon the shoulders of its predecessors, and the fair perspectives that are now opening before you are largely the creation of those who have gone before you. It is therefore reasonable to think that anyone who has spent a long professional life in medicine must have something to hand on—however small or modest.*
>
> Sir F.M.R. Walshe, *Canadian Medical Association Journal*
> 1952;67:395.

Have you ever thought: "I have learned a lot in medical school and specialty training (and perhaps in practice). Wouldn't it be great to teach students and residents what I know? Maybe I could even do some research. I wonder what a teaching career is really like. Might a career in academic medicine be right for me?"

THE JOY OF TEACHING

"Doctor Taylor, I made the diagnosis! His symptoms were just what you described in class." Out of breath from running across the courtyard outside the cafeteria, this medical student, Jennifer, couldn't wait to tell me about her diagnostic triumph.

Every 6 weeks I teach a small-group seminar for third-year medical students about the diagnosis and management of headaches. In the session, we spend about 5 or 10 minutes discussing cluster headache. A few weeks earlier, Jennifer had been part of my seminar group. Subsequently, as part of the clerkship, she had been seeing patients in the office of a community family physician, when a young man came in with a history of a series of terrible headaches that had been prompting him to visit the emergency room, where he had received various injections of pain-killers, but no definitive diagnosis.

Jennifer had interviewed the patient prior to his seeing the doctor. When he told of his recent series of once-daily headaches and a similar series about 9 months ago, Jennifer had one of these "Aha!" moments that, regrettably, clinicians experience all too rarely. She asked some more questions, everything fit, and she presented the patient to her preceptor with a tentative diagnosis of cluster headache. Of course, she was correct, and for the patient, it was the initial identification of the problem.

No wonder Jennifer was excited and couldn't wait to tell me about it.

For the academic clinician involved in teaching medical students and residents, this sort of experience is a highlight that you will recall happily for a long time. Teaching is why most of us chose academic careers.

One of our contributors, who entered academic medicine soon after residency, writes, "I grew up wanting to be a teacher, but I didn't believe that I could teach medicine until early in my residency. From that point, it was just a matter of choosing between practice-based teaching, residency-based teaching, or medical school–based teaching."

Another contributor is a radiologist who made the move to academic medicine after three decades in successful private practice. When asked why, he replies, "I wanted to do some teaching." This is a common response by our book's contributors, but there can be other reasons as well. Later he adds, "Also, I wanted to give something back to medicine."

But there is more to academic medicine than teaching. Teaching is definitely part of what you do but may be a small part of your daily activities. There will also be clinical care, probably some administration, and the opportunity for research and scholarship. While doing this, you should also learn about the organizational dynamics of the academic medical center, including the cultural expectations, the hierarchy of power, and the unspoken rules. I tell you much of this in the pages to come—but not all. When it comes to teaching skills, research, medical writing, and getting grants, there is way too much for this single volume; many books and articles have been written on these topics, and I will provide tables listing some of my favorite resources.

At this point, I think it is important to examine the phrase I will use in the book to describe the clinician who chooses an academic career: the *academic clinician*. And that will also take me, early in the book, to an area of controversy.

THE ACADEMIC CLINICIAN

Before I began writing this book, I thought a great deal about what I will call us—patient-care-oriented physicians who work in academic medical centers where there is the opportunity to teach, administer programs, do research, and write for publication. In fact, there is more than the opportunity; excellence in one or more of the nonclinical parts of the job is the key to advancement and "academic success."

Currently, a number of terms are used. Two terms you will hear are "clinician-educators" and "clinician-teachers." The former is most commonly used. Branch and colleagues use the terms interchangeably.[1] Over the past 10 to 15 years, academic medical centers (AMCs) have established clinician-educator faculty positions, which now constitute an entry-level academic job for many young physicians.

Branch and colleagues state that, "Although no consensus exists, the essence of all definitions includes the concept of a superior clinician, who is also a dedicated teacher."[1] This is the academic rationale. However, on an economic basis, the clinician-educator positions were established because AMCs needed clinicians to generate income that would support the institution in the face of decreasing federal and state funding for education and for hospital care of the needy. Thus, clinician-educators are filling an important need but are not necessarily highly respected in the institution. When the status of the clinician-educator is contrasted with the status of research-oriented faculty, the reality of the two-tiered academic system becomes, in the jargon of Wall Street, transparent.

The most flagrant evidence of the status differential becomes evident when we consider the award of tenure and promotion in rank. Tenure, the more-or-less guarantee of job security, is a time-honored academic reward. An appointment as a clinician-educator, with scant expectation of participating in scholarly activity, offers inherent obstacles to promotion and tenure. According to Levinson and Rubenstein: "Most often, these new tracks did not offer the possibility of tenure, partly because of the reluctance of academic institutions to make long-term financial commitments to faculty members with primarily clinical and teaching responsibilities."[2]

As far as promotion is concerned, the academic medical centers have done a cautious soft-shoe dance. Most medical schools have established special criteria for promotion of clinician-educators.[3] However, in the process, the institutions have added adjectives such as "clinical" to the designation of rank. Thus, instead of becoming an associate professor, one might be a "clinical associate professor," and we all know that this descriptor connotes lower scholarly achievement. (See Chapters 2 and 3 for more about the academic promotion process.)

In 1999, Levinson and Rubenstein recommended that the promotion requirement of a regional or national reputation be eliminated for clinician-educators. They also wrote, "Second, the requirement of publication in peer-reviewed journals should be eliminated."[2] They go on to state that, "Academic institutions should find new and creative ways to evaluate clinician-educators' teaching abilities and clinical excellence."[2] But, to me, this seems to perpetuate the two-tiered system.

Apparently, their proposed changes did not entirely satisfy Levinson and Rubenstein, either. The next year, writing in the journal *Academic Medicine*, they proposed "the development of a new faculty position, a 'clinician-educator-researcher' to foster the scholarship of discovery in medical education and clinical practice." This idea was appealing until I read on to find that the authors recommend that these physicians "receive advanced Master's or PhD-level training in the area of education." They go on to recommend that,

"Subsequent to such training, AMCs will need to support these faculty members, who will need to devote more than 75% of their effort to research endeavors concerning education or clinical care, similar to the effort of faculty conducting basic biomedical research."[4] I was on board until the proposed requirements for advanced degrees and 75% research effort. Also, "clinician-educator-researcher" has too many syllables for me. The phrase feels unwieldy.

For the rest of this book, I will use the term "academic clinician." It means what I wish Levinson and Rubinstein had proposed. In the pages to come, "academic clinician" describes a physician who treats sick people, teaches residents and students, and engages in scholarly activity—even if the three activities are not in equal balance.

Some have called this the "triple-threat academician," an allusion to the football player who can run, pass, and kick the ball. In today's specialized world, many medical faculty members choose not to be triple-threat and to emphasize a single facet of their career to the virtual extinction of the others. And many of these academicians become quite successful developing only one narrowly focused academic ability, usually research. In fact, some say that the triple-threat academician is now an anachronism. I believe that this might have been true when research ruled in AMCs, when teaching and clinical care were less valued. But today, with the increasing need for clinical income, AMCs are recruiting and hiring clinicians. We just need to find ways to help these newly hired clinicians achieve first-class academic status.

I am aware that I am not the first to use the term "academic clinician." For example the University of Pennsylvania School of Medicine uses the term to describe full-time untenured appointments with the word "clinical" added to designation of faculty rank. Johns Hopkins has "academic clinicians." I am sure some other AMCs also do.

I will deal later with how the academic clinician fits into the academic milieu, achieves appropriate balance, focuses his or her energies, gets promoted, and, who knows, maybe attains tenure. First, I will examine the decision to become an academic clinician.

BECOMING AN ACADEMIC CLINICIAN

It is time to leave semantics and controversy and to be practical. If you are now a medical student, resident, fellow, or practicing physician reading this page, I assume that you are considering (or perhaps have already made) a career-defining decision. If you are a newly minted junior faculty member, you have embarked on a transformational journey.

The Career Decision

The decision to seek an academic career is, in many ways, like choosing your medical specialty. In medical school, you and I pondered, "Shall I become a pediatrician, pathologist, or neurosurgeon?" First of all, there is the consideration of what you will give up: If you are a medical student and you choose to become, for example, an internist, you give up maternity care forever. If you become a psychiatrist, you forsake abdominal surgery. And, of course, each specialty has its own "personality profile," culture, and values.[5]

Choosing an academic career pathway also has profound implications for your life. An ill-informed decision will leave you frustrated every day at work. If you enter private practice, government service, military medicine, or any of several nonacademic careers, you might do a little teaching in your office and perhaps write a paper or two, but teaching and discovery will not be part of your "job description." On the other hand, if you choose to be an academic clinician, you forsake the autonomy you might enjoy with small group practice, in which you have some control of your scope of practice, equipment purchases, and even personnel hiring decisions. For example, in many AMCs the nurses and receptionists in the clinics work for the hospital and not for the clinicians; the latter have little say in staffing levels, the skills of those hired, and even in what hours nurses work. For residents and fellows entering academic medicine, limitations such as these may seem insignificant. For physicians who have had a taste of private practice independence, losing the ability to select your nurse co-workers, control your patient scheduling, or even decide on what time you begin and end the workday can be a *big issue*.

At this time, let us examine what you really have in mind when you become an academic clinician. What is your dream? Do you see yourself being part of a patient care team that deals with the difficult cases referred from community hospitals to the AMC? This is not an unrealistic expectation. Do you see yourself as the doctor who serves the under-served, the beacon of hope for those who cannot pay for care? If this is your vision, then be sure that it is consistent with the mission of the AMC. (Of course, you can, as in private practice, serve the underserved during off-duty hours.) Do you see yourself spending your days sharing your accumulated wisdom with eager students? Some of this will happen but generally not as much as you might imagine. Instances of grateful feedback as I had from Jennifer (see the beginning of this chapter) don't occur daily. You may even see yourself performing research and writing impor-tant papers that receive critical acclaim. This is possible but will require learning some skills that they did not teach us in medical school.

One important caution: Beware of career choices seeking to emulate an attractive role model. You—as a sensitive, process-oriented medical student who likes spending time with your family and who really didn't like the messiness of procedures during your surgical rotation—would not choose cardiothoracic surgery as a specialty just because you spent time with a very charismatic and talented heart surgeon. A similar situation can happen in academics. You may have made the best possible specialty choice and are now in a psy-chiatry residency or gastroenterology fellowship. Your lead instructor and mentor is an academician who is seen as a rising star in his specialty. He invites you to apply for the faculty position that is now available. Should you do so?

Remember that what is right for one person may not be right for you. Although you may admire your teacher and mentor in academics, do not confuse admiration with solid decision-making. In career decisions, remember this: We cli-nicians who love what we do are always seeking to clone ourselves. I am sad to report that in this quest for cloning, we medical educators often guide medical students into specialties for which they are temperamentally unsuited. Also, we sometimes encourage academic careers for some who would be better advised to enter private practice.

Learning About Life in Academia

Whatever your fantasy about life as an academician, you should talk to many who have walked the path before you. Spend time with both neophyte and seasoned faculty. Ask them about their lives in academia and especially about what they might not tell you unless asked. Ask the questions that I am going to describe next.

In preparing this book, I sought the participation of 20 academic physicians in a variety of specialties and academic settings. I asked them to respond to 10 open-ended questions, and I used the answers to help prepare this book. I include responses as examples throughout the pages that follow and in a number of the tables. Here are the questions and, in parentheses, the book chapters where responses chiefly appear:

Questions Answered by Contributors (and Chapters Where Responses Will Be Included)

- Tell about your decision to choose an academic medicine career. (1)
- How has your life changed since becoming an "academic clinician?" (1)
- What do you like about being an academic clinician? What don't you like? (2)
- What have been the surprises, pleasant and unpleasant, about your academic job? (2)
- What are important unwritten rules about academia? (3)
- How did you find your first academic position? (4)
- Have you had a mentor and, if so, how has that person influenced your career? (8)
- If you could do one thing differently in your career, what would it be? (9)
- What advice would you give the new academic clinician? (10)

■ Will you please tell an anecdote—a story that is meaningful to you—about your experience in academic medicine? (10)

Why Choose an Academic Career?

Whenever considering a career change, you should always
ask, "Am I changing to follow a dream *or* am I trying to
escape a bad situation?" I earnestly hope that all who seek
careers as academic clinicians are following their vision of
the best career path and the best opportunity to serve
humanity.

Table 1.1 tells some general reasons why we choose academic medical careers. Some are positive reasons; some are
not. On the plus side, seeking a teaching role, yearning for
the opportunity to seek new knowledge, or looking for a
greater intellectual challenge are all reasons I find reassur-
ing. The reasons in the "worrisome" column should arouse
concern.

Residents and fellows might consider academics as a way
to avoid the "business of medicine" or might even uncon-
sciously seek to prolong the adolescence of being a learner.
The "avoidance" reasons are not a firm foundation for an
academic career. Physicians who enter academics to escape
a current conflict with partners, a chaotic practice situation,
or a messy divorce should perhaps consider other options.

TABLE 1.1. Seeking an academic career: Positive reasons and worrisome
reasons

Positive reasons	Worrisome reasons
Wanting to teach students and residents	Seeking to escape a difficult practice or personal situation
Wanting the intellectual enrichment of the academic life	Becoming tired of hard work and night call
Seeking the diversity of activities that is found in academic medicine	Looking for an escape from patient care
Wishing to do research and write	Searching for a less stressful life
Looking for a new professional challenge	Wanting to earn a high income

Some older physicians will seek academic life as a way to "retire into teaching"; such a move is unfair to learners, who deserve our best efforts at all times.

The new academician from community practice who aims to get away from a hectic schedule may be disappointed to learn that, whereas in private practice one has only to attend to patient care, the academic clinician finds responsibilities in the three major spheres of clinical practice, teaching, and scholarship. It is common for new academicians to say "yes" to far too many opportunities and soon feel scattered and overwhelmed. So much for avoiding a busy schedule and stressful professional life.

And in case there is any question about the pay, an academic medical career is seldom a ticket to the Lifestyle of the Rich and Famous. A few academicians, generally surgeons who work very hard, become wealthy. Most academic physicians find that they must earn most or all of their own salaries while also earning enough to underwrite the time spent teaching. Finding funding support for research time is a special issue that I will discuss in Chapter 6. Do not expect an academic institution to support your research for more than a short time, if at all.

A survey of physicians identified the top 10 reasons physicians leave their current job.[6] The top reason given was the need for a higher salary. Seeking better compensation may be a valid justification for leaving a job, but it is a very poor reason to seek a position at an academic medical center.

The Decision

I asked our contributors to, "Tell about your decision to choose an academic medicine career." Here are some of the responses:

■ "I have wanted to teach ever since I was toilet trained. . . ."
■ "Contrary to your caution about emulating a charismatic mentor, my decision came when, fresh out of college, I stumbled into an opportunity as an American Heart Association Fellow that allowed me to work with

TABLE 1.2. Books, articles, and Web sites where you can learn more about academic medical careers

Books
Bland CJ, Schmitz CC, Stritter FT, Henry RC, Aluise JJ. Successful faculty in academic medicine: essential skills and how to acquire them. New York: Springer, 1990.

Boice R. Advice for new faculty members. Needham Heights, MA: Allyn and Bacon, 2000.

Douglas KC, Hosokawa MC, Lawler FH. A practical guide to clinical teaching in medicine. New York: Springer, 1988.

McCabe LRB, McCabe ER. How to succeed in academics. New York: Academic Press, 2000. (This is a short [147 page] book on general academic skills: grant applications, leadership, lecturing. But there is nothing specific about academic medicine.)

Schwenk TL, Whitman N. The physician as teacher. Baltimore: Williams & Wilkins, 1987.

Scott M. Planning for a successful career transition: the physician's guide to managing career change. Chicago: American Medical Association, 1999.

Articles
Jones RF, Gold JS. The present and future of appointment, tenure, and compensation policies for medical school clinical faculty. Acad Med 2001;76:993–1004.

McGuire LK, Bergen MR, Polan ML. Career advancement for women faculty in a U.S. school of medicine: perceived needs. Acad Med 2004;79:319–325.

McLennan G. Is the master clinician dead? Acad Med 2001;76:617–619.

Levinson W, Rubenstein A. Integrating clinician-educators into academic medical centers: challenges and potential solutions. Acad Med 2000;75:906–912.

Web sites
Academic Physician and Scientist: available at http://www.acphysci.com/aps/app/.

The Association of American Medical Colleges: available at http://www.aamc.org/.

The Accreditation Council on Graduate Medical Education: available at http://www.acgme.org/.

The Riley Guide (to job listings in health care and medical fields): available at http://www.rileyguide.com/health.html/.

an inspiring physician. Knowing next to nothing about a career in academic medicine (and obviously having little insight about my own values and motivations), seeing this individual enjoying challenging rewards as a clinician, teacher, researcher, and activist was mesmerizing. I remember thinking I wanted a job exactly like his!"

■ "The primary reason I chose academics was to create a balance in my career that would allow me to remain clinically active and simultaneously participate in basic science and clinical research related to the care of my patients. My job is ego gratifying, high energy, and intellectually stimulating, all of which are additive to the day-in and day-out work of an orthopedic surgeon."

■ "I had a typical midlife crisis, decided I was in a rut, and left private practice mostly in search of a change and to prove to myself that I could still change."

■ "I took an American College of Physician Executives course on Career Choices. Academic medicine met most of my goals of teaching, practicing medicine, and using my administrative skills."

■ "My decision to become an academic was based on factors other than a large amount of intellectual curiosity, or an overwhelming desire to teach at the time I was hired. A big factor was a personality match with the department chairman. I trusted and admired the man."

■ "I love teaching, and being able to make an impact on the next generation of physicians is very satisfying. Also, I entered academics in order to have some influence on reform of our health care system and medical education."

MYTHS ABOUT ACADEMIC CAREERS

What We Do All Day

One day I was speaking with one of my colleagues in community practice, and I mentioned a difficult diagnosis I was facing with one of my patients in the hospital. My physician colleague asked, incredulously, "Do mean that you guys see patients?" He, and many like him, believed that we spent our time teaching, doing some research, traveling to medical meetings, and thinking deep thoughts—but no actual patient care.

In fact, all academicians, except those fully funded on research grants, must see patients to generate most or all or their salaries. In the next chapter, I will tell some detail about how salaries are determined. Here I will tell you now that one of the eye-opening facts I learned after moving from private practice to academic medicine is that there is no pot of money available to pay your salary year after year. What your academic appointment gets you—and your department—is a "hunting license" to go out and search for your salary support through practice income or grants.

More Curious Myths About Academia

The belief that academic clinicians do not see patients is just one of several myths that exist about academic careers. Here are some more:

Myth: The Skills That Make You a Successful Practitioner Are Just What Are Needed for Success in Academic Medicine

In academia, being a good clinician is not enough. I entered academic medicine with, I modestly believe, excellent clinical practice skills. In my first years on faculty, I received several resident teaching awards based on my patient care abilities that I brought from private practice. Residents are a tough audience and do not give such awards frivolously. But I found that I was sadly lacking in other academic survival skills.

Let's talk about management decisions, for example. In my private solo office, I had been the unquestioned chief. Policies were what I decided. Changes were rarely "negotiated." I set the work hours, salaries, and even how the telephone would be answered. But upon entering academic medicine, I discovered that almost every decision, however minor it might seem, affected others who demanded a voice. If I wanted to see two more patients each half day, I needed to discuss this with the office manager, scheduler, and nurses. Once when I announced a plan to have a research assistant interview patients in the waiting room (this was, of course, pre-HIPAA), I nearly caused a revolt.

Unions, when they get involved, generally make the problem more complex. Once our academic practice had a successful year financially and we decided to give a bonus to our office staff. Then the employee union learned of our intention. "No, you can't give a bonus to employees in your clinic. Other clinics in the medical center are not doing so, and therefore it would be unfair for your staff to receive bonuses." Incredible, but true!

Myth: Medical Schools Seek and Reward Great Teachers

Medical students and residents appreciate dedicated and energetic teachers. However, of the three main missions of the AMC—clinical care, teaching, and scholarship—guess which one brings in little or no funding. The answer is, of course, teaching. For this reason, medical school departments tend to lose great teachers and retain successful clinicians, researchers, and grant writers who can bring in salary support. The latter group may not be the best teachers and, in fact, may be reluctant educators.

A study from one academic medical center looked at recipients of a "Teacher of the Year" award in a department of internal medicine.[7] The researchers found that teaching award winners left the department sooner than those who did not receive the award, even after adjustment for age, rank, and career track.

Myth: Your Job Description Includes a Lot of Time to Think, Do Research, and Write

If much of your time is spent earning your salary, then when do you do your creative thinking, research, and writing? The candid answer: For most academicians, scholarly work is done weekends and evenings. In fact, it is now Saturday morning as I type these words. Over the years, some young faculty members have become angry when I have told them about the need to do scholarly work on personal time. But with the many clinical, teaching, and administrative duties that compete for time during work hours, there is never enough time for scholarship. It works out as follows: patients cannot be neglected, student and resident teaching obligations must be met, and administrative tasks require timely attention. Scholarly projects just keep being moved to the bottom of the pile at work. This happens over and over until you see the light and begin to take the research study or writing project home for the weekend.

Myth: You Will End Each Workday by 5 p.m.

This is a cruel joke. The truth is that, with the array of competing obligations faced by the academician, your workday may actually be longer in a teaching setting than in private practice. Only the most compulsively well organized or the most slothful get out the door by 5 p.m. Furthermore, in AMCs there are many events that occur in the evening: administrative meetings, faculty social events, resident and student activities, and more.

Yes, you can declare that your evenings and weekends are your own and refuse participation in all after-hours activities. This is, however, a bad career move. It quickly marks you as one who is really not committed to the department and institution, and this perception of your being "not committed" becomes reflected in opportunities that might have been yours being passed to others.

Myth: You Can Plan on a Funded Sabbatical Every Seventh Year

This may be true at a medical school somewhere in the United States, but I don't know what school that is. With the economic squeeze on AMCs today. the opportunities for sabbatical time are becoming increasingly limited.

A sabbatical is still a possibility at many institutions under certain circumstances: First of all, there probably won't be full funding for your time away. The responsibility for paying you any salary at all will probably fall to your department, which is likely to be having trouble making its annual payroll as it is.

If you wish a sabbatical experience, be prepared to present a compelling case as to how your time will be spent doing something that will ultimately benefit the institution. This means that, after the sabbatical, you should plan to return with a fundable grant proposal, a new and much-needed clinical skill, or the high probability of launching a new (and, again, fundable) research endeavor. Coming back from a sabbatical feeling renewed and energized is no longer enough.

Myth: Working in an AMC Offers More Job Security Than Private Practice

This is quaint legend about academia. Unless you hold a tenured position, you are vulnerable, and even tenured faculty can see funding disappear (see Chapter 3). If you do not have tenure, you are likely to be on a year-to-year contract. Each year, at the anniversary of your hiring, your chair may decide not to renew your contract.

IMPORTANT QUESTIONS TO BE ANSWERED

If I haven't scared you away by now, there are other important questions to be answered. The answers concern what you need to know and how you think and feel. Here are some of these questions.

Am I Ready for Academic Life?

Only you can decide that you are temperamentally suited to life as an academic clinician. The means that you must take a hard look at yourself.

Favorable Traits

You may be ready and might even be quite successful in academic medicine if you possess the following traits:

- Flexibility—the ability to adapt to new situations. Remember that in the theory of evolution, the species that survived were not the strongest or fiercest but those who could adapt to change.
- Vigor—a high level of energy is required to meet the challenges of multiple responsibilities in the domains of clinical care, teaching, scholarship, administration, mentorship, and more.

- Curiosity—because wondering "Why?" is the basis of scholarship, as I will discuss later in Chapters 5 and 6.
- Self-confidence—which is needed to hold your own in meetings, to weather criticism of your teaching, and to withstand disagreement with your scholarly opinions.
- Integrity—to compel you to make the right decisions, even in difficult circumstances. Right, but tough, decisions might include disciplining the poorly performing resident, failing the student who refuses to show up for class, telling a colleague that he made a clinical error, or informing a colleague that she has reached unjustified conclusions in a paper she has written.

Unfavorable Traits

You may want to take a long time deciding on an academic career if you have the following personal traits:

- Independence—connoting a fierce tendency to work best alone. This is an excellent trait for writers, hermits, and physicians in solo practice. It is not helpful in academic medicine, when you work side by side with others in almost all settings. Sometimes, very successful clinicians enter an academic setting with the idea that they can practice exactly as they did in the private world. They eventually—and painfully—learn that an academic group practice must be one in which all physicians conform to agreed-upon rules of how the practice will be conducted.
- Selfishness—thinking of your own interests before those of others. The academic clinician must often put learners or other faculty first. A physician who is seen as always out for his or her own interests is soon shut out of research proposals, writing projects, event planning and new opportunities.
- Rigidity—the inability to adapt to the needs of others and to the changes about you will predict a short academic career. The cry of the rigid physician is, "I don't care what the group decides. I won't do it that way!" This attitude—in relation to patient care, teaching methods, or research planning—is poison to effective group decision-making and will not long be tolerated by colleagues.

How Will My Life Change as an Academic Clinician?

Medical Students, Residents, and Fellows

If you are a student, resident, or fellow, your life will almost certainly improve. You will have more authority, respect, and pay. You will probably have a more favorable night and weekend call schedule, especially because residents and fellows (which you were just recently) will take care of much routine after-hours work; you will be contacted for "important problems." You will even have an office, although it may be shared with others. You will also have some newly acquired expectations to teach and engage in scholarship.

Practicing Physicians

If you are a practicing physician entering academic medicine, I believe that the changes will be more profound than those experienced by residents and fellows moving directly to academic careers. You, the practicing doctor who has been recruited to academics because of your patient-care skills, will need to fit into the academic mold in the many ways described in this book. The impact will vary directly with your years away from medical school and residency.

On balance, you will bring to the AMC your knowledge of efficient practice models, real-world clinical experience, and a patient-centered ethic.

What the Contributors Report

I asked our book's contributors to tell, "How has your life changed since becoming an academic clinician?" In reading the responses below, keep in mind that the contributors represent a broad spectrum of specialties, academic experience, and pathways to their current careers. With that said, here are what I consider the most helpful responses (with a few editorial comments in italic):

■ "I am challenged daily with learners (and colleagues) from every level of training. This challenge has given me the passion to stay current, more so than I believe I might in private practice."

■ "I was amazed at how much time was spent in meetings. As a resident and fellow, we had some teaching seminars and grand rounds, but as a new academic doctor, I have more meetings than I ever imagined. I guess the meetings are important, but they get me behind on seeing my patients and getting my chart work done." (*The respondent is a gastroenterologist in his second year of an academic position.*)

■ "I now have a much more scheduled lifestyle. It is easier clinically, although clinical challenges are still there and I'm sure will be until I retire. I'm on tenure track and so there is the pressure of getting grants and publishing. But I get home at 6 p.m. instead of 9 p.m., and patients never call me at home now, as they frequently did when I was in private practice." (*Yes, this response seems at odds with the third myth described above. No two academic jobs are alike, and a difference of opinion is accepted in academics.*)

■ "Life is more structured with dedicated teaching and research time. Specific goals can be identified and met."

■ "The intellectual stimulation is great, and having close friends and colleagues from around the country is very rewarding."

■ "I read more yet still feel like I never quite know my field as well as I should. I'm a bit rusty in some of my clinical skills (starting IVs, doing lumbar punctures, attending deliveries), because house staff do most of those."

■ "I've spent all of my professional life in academic medicine. As I've learned how things work in the academic environment, I've had an easier time knowing how to react. But the overall attraction of creating a learning environment has been a constant. As a department chair, I now simply do this for faculty instead of just for residents and students."

■ "Working closely with residents and students keeps one on one's toes and up to date."

Do I Know as Much as I Need to Know About the Academic Career I Am Considering?

The answer to this question will, of course, always be "no." After 27 years in academic medicine, I don't know all there is to know. But I keep trying to learn and so should you.

In conversations with junior faculty members, I find that what they wished they had known more about falls into two large categories. The first category is somewhat theoretical; it concerns the true pluses and minuses of academic life and the surprises new faculty members encounter. The second category of I-wish-I-had-known items is more practical and is focused on job descriptions, faculty tracks and ranks, and compensation issues.

These two categories of topics are covered in Chapter 2.

REFERENCES

1. Branch WT, Kroenke K, Levinson W. The clinician-educator: present and future roles. J Gen Int Med 1997;12(Suppl. 2): S1–S4.
2. Levinson W, Rubenstein. Mission critical—integrating clinician-educators into academic medical centers. N Engl J Med 1999;341:840–843.
3. Jones RF, Gold JS. Faculty appointment and tenure policies in medical schools. Acad Med 1998;73:212–219.
4. Levinson W, Rubenstein. Integrating clinician-educators into academic medical centers: challenges and potential solutions. Acad Med 2000;75:906–912.
5. Taylor AD. How to choose a medical specialty, 4th ed. Philadelphia: WB Saunders, 2003.
6. Abdo W, Broxterman MP. Why physicians change jobs: survey shows salary tops the list. Physicians Practice 2004;14(7):34.
7. Aucott JC, Como J, Aron DC. Teaching awards and departmental longevity: is award-winning the "kiss of death" in an academic department of medicine? Perspect Biol Med 1999; 42:280–287.

2

About an Academic Career

Welcome to Chapter 2. In the first chapter, I discussed the process of deciding on an academic career. You will make the best decision only if you know as much as possible about the job you will be doing and the setting in which you will be working. This chapter tells about faculty positions, and Chapter 3 describes the setting—the academic medical center (AMC).

In this chapter, I will present two types of data. One type is subjective and experiential data; the chapter will begin with a section on "How Clinicians Feel About Their Academic Careers" and end with "Surprises Reported by Academic Clinicians." The other type of data is more objective—explanations of academic job descriptions, faculty tracks and ranks, salary compensation, and gender and ethnic/racial issues in academic careers.

HOW CLINICIANS FEEL ABOUT THEIR ACADEMIC CAREERS

"A man's happiness is to do a man's true work," wrote Marcus Aurelius (*Meditations* VIII.xxvi). For some of us, being an academic clinician is our "true work." I have been known to say that I have so much fun at work that I felt guilty taking a paycheck at the end of the month. If you are temperamentally suited to an academic career and are successful in landing the job that is right for you, you will enjoy almost every day at work. Well, most of every day. There are some aspects of an academic job—such as telling a student that he or she is not fulfilling expectations—that are never fun.

What Contributors Like About Their Jobs

As I prepared notes for this book, I asked academicians in various specialties what they liked and what they didn't like about their jobs. To put some order to the replies, I have arranged them by categories. Some of the responses that follow may resonate with you. Others may not. In fact, what excites one clinician about his or her job may be just what another finds tedious. Here is what our contributors replied when asked, "What do you like about being an academic clinician?"

Clinical Practice

■ "At the medical center we get to see the difficult cases, the problems that can't be handled at the smaller community hospitals. Last night I admitted a young woman who was very toxic, with high fever and delirium. She had been camping with friends in the mountains, which means possible exposure to ticks, mosquitos, and who knows what else. No one else in the group had any illness at all. We are in the process of figuring out the diagnosis while treating her empirically. And, in managing this problem, I have all the resources of the medical center at my disposal."

■ "I enjoy the opportunity to think about the cases I see and have intelligent discussions about the differential diagnoses, instead of a factory-type environment where the dollar is the bottom line."

■ "What I like best of all is working with clinicians in all the different specialties. If I need to consult a pediatric neurologist, one is available. If my patient requires a consultation with a dermatopathologist, there is one on staff."

■ "Whenever the community hospital has a really interesting case, they are likely to send the patient here [to the AMC]."

Education

■ "Perhaps the greatest lure for me is the opportunity—and the privilege—to teach."

■ "Working with students and residents is the best part of my day. I especially like my time with students. They are idealistic and open-minded. I feel that I can really make a difference in how they think about medicine."

■ "Being around young enthusiastic students who are starting out."

Scholarship

■ "I like the sense that what I do on a daily basis may extend beyond the immediate health care needs of individuals and families and may ultimately affect whole communities and populations."

■ "For me, the most fun is helping a resident or a young faculty member with a research project. The challenge is to take a general idea and develop a testable hypothesis. Then we figure out a way to answer the questions we have framed. I really enjoy this type of intellectual challenge, which would not be available to me in private practice."

Administration

■ "Maybe I have a sick mind, but I really enjoy working on quality assurance. I lead our department's quality assurance effort, which seeks the best possible care for our patients. We focus on ways to apply evidence-based medicine in our clinics, and I think that what I do helps all our clinicians practice up-to-date, patient-friendly medicine."

Career and Lifestyle

■ "In a word, variety."

■ "I can work part time."

■ "Our medical school has an excellent office of faculty development. The assistant dean for faculty development and her staff work with all departments to present opportunities for us to enhance our pedagogical skills. We recently had a seminar on 'How to Lead a Small Group Discussion.' I learned several things I could do better. I believe that the faculty development program is helping me do my job better and is certainly teaching me things I didn't learn in medical school."

■ "Travel. My academic job gives me the chance to attend—and present papers at—meetings in the U.S. and sometimes abroad. If I were in private practice, I would not have this opportunity. I probably wouldn't be invited as an 'expert' to speak and I would not have the travel funds that my institution provides.

■ "I find that I have more dependable personal time. Sure, I have some evening events that I have to attend. But when night call comes along, the residents take the first call, and I am consulted only for the complicated problems. Also, with a large faculty, we are able to spread the night call around. One person being on vacation is not the problem it might be in a small private practice."

■ "I like flexibility and challenges of using my skills as a teacher, administrator, leader, and clinician."

■ "With conferences, students, and residents around, every day is a learning experience."

■ "I feel very lucky that I have the position that I had wanted since being in medical school. I like the diverse roles of clinical responsibilities, teaching and directing courses, and research. I also enjoy leadership roles in two national organizations. The schedule in academic medicine also gives some flexibility, which has supported the survival of my two-career family."

■ "I like the environment of innovation and creativity. I like the scholarly environment and the fact that I learn new things every day. And I love the challenge of working with really smart and highly motivated people."

What Contributors Don't Like About Their Jobs

Thoreau said, "Most men would feel insulted if it were proposed to employ them in throwing stones over a wall and then in throwing them back, merely that they might earn their wages. But many are no more worthily employed now." (Henry David Thoreau, *Life Without Principle*, 1863.) Although no academician is likely to think of his or her job as being the pointless, repetitive activity Thoreau describes, it is true that not every minute of every day is a peak experience. Here are some criticisms reported by clinicians when asked, "What don't you like about your academic job?"

Clinical Practice

■ "One thing I don't like about academic medicine is having less clinical time than my colleagues in private practice."

■ "I feel like I am pressured to give away all the interesting cases. Sure, it is nice to have all the super-specialized docs around, but whenever there is a really fascinating case, they swoop in and claim it as their 'turf.' I feel that if I were in community practice, I would be in more control of what cases I manage and when to refer to others."

■ "I don't like the financial squeeze we face as clinicians, having difficulty supporting the academic enterprise with clinical dollars."

■ "I miss the close personal relationships with patients."

■ "There is always someone looking over my shoulder. There are coders, the quality assurance committee, the residents, etc. Even nurses feel free to write up complaints about my care. Sometimes I get a little tired of the 'Big Brother is watching you' feeling of the medical center."

Education

■ "Frankly, sometimes the residents and even the medical students seem disrespectful of patients. Something seems to happen about the third year of medical school that changes them from idealistic, caring individuals into pessimistic, disparaging persons. Faculty describe this as the transition from the 'pre-cynical' to the 'cynical' years of medical school."

■ "I don't like that although academic medicine says it values good teaching, rewards and promotions are biased toward bringing in research dollars."

Scholarship

■ "There is definitely pressure for me to do research and write, but I am not interested in these areas. I really just want to see patients and provide excellent clinical care. I wish my department chair would understand this and stop trying to make me into something I'm not—a research scientist."

■ "Getting grant reviews back where it is obvious the reviewer didn't know the territory."

Administration

■ I don't like the arcane politics of an academic health center, and I'm not convinced it is well run from a business standpoint."

■ "Administrative tasks can get to be burdensome, especially in a very large institution where the politics are quite intricate."

■ "Fund-raising responsibility."

■ "I never expected to find that the job involved so many meetings. When I took the job, I knew that I would see patients, teach, and maybe write a little. But yesterday, I was in two meetings, and I had a 5 p.m. meeting the day before. Tomorrow there is a 90-minute meeting that begins at 7 a.m., and this causes problems with my child's day care. If it weren't for the meetings, this would be a great job."

■ "I don't like the fact that our medical college has more people in place that can slow or stop implementation of new ideas than it has people who will innovate."

Career and Lifestyle

■ "I think the hours are longer."

■ "There are endless demands on my time. It can be very hard to say 'no' to a colleague or supervisor, especially at the beginning of an academic career."

■ "Everyone is saying to 'Be a leader.' But no one taught me leadership skills in medical school or residency, and there is no leadership training in my institution. So I am reading some books and trying to figure things out on my own. In the meantime, I keep being put in charge of task forces and committees, where I learn by trial and error."

■ "The travel is getting me down. In the beginning I liked to go to meetings and give lectures. But now I am tired of being away from home, and yet I know that I must establish my national reputation if I am ever going to be promoted.

- "I don't like the hierarchy, the lack of democracy. We used to vote on everything in practice. It was a democracy. This [academic medicine] is more like the military. Autocratic. Everything is decided by the dean and the chair."
- "A lot of folks in academic medicine are really full of themselves and take themselves too seriously, sometimes."

About Realistic Expectations

Recently, a colleague received an e-mail message and sent it on to me. The author is a pediatrician in private practice seeking an academic job. After lamenting increased professional liability premiums, poor reimbursement, and 5- to 10-minute visits, the physician continues:

> I remember fondly the staff at the my medical school and how they supported the students. I now believe that even though I may miss some aspects of direct patient care, moving to a role that supports others to pursue a medical career would be very satisfying. That is why I am writing to inquire where there are any employment opportunities. . . .

This physician hopes to enter academics and apparently wants a job with no direct patient care and that instead involves only teaching and student counseling.

I believe that the job-seeking pediatrician needs a much better understanding of what an academic career really involves. This understanding may logically begin with the academic job description.

THE ACADEMIC JOB DESCRIPTION

If you and an academic department enter into discussion about an academic job, there exists a formal description of the position's title, duties, and responsibilities. You may see the position description posted on a bulletin board or on the Web. Or you may first encounter it later in the recruitment process. If you are considering a faculty opening, it is a good idea to request a copy of the position description if one does not arrive with the first packet of information.

Contents of the Academic Position Description

Academic job descriptions, although often quite concise, will usually contain the following elements:

Position Title

This describes the job you are discussing. It may be titled "Clinician-Educator" or "Clinician-Teacher," which suggests an entry-level position. Farther up the power ladder are position titles such as "Associate Clinic Director," "Director of Research," "Residency Director," or even "Department Chair."

Salary Range

This tells the funds available for the position, depending on the qualifications of the applicant.

Full-Time Equivalent (FTE)

This is pedagogical jargon for the amount of time allocated to the job. An FTE of 1.0 means a full-time job; 0.5 FTE is a half-time job. In many institutions, 0.5 FTE is the cutoff for receiving fringe benefits, which is a very important part of the discussion (see Chapter 4).

Dates

Dates you might see include the date the job opening was first posted, closing date for applications, and starting date for the position.

Responsibilities

This is the key part of the position description. Look for statements in four categories, which may or may not be identified by a breakdown of the total FTE into each area:

■ Clinical responsibilities: This section describes the patient care you will be expected to provide and may include specific language about what the person filling the job will do in clinic, hospital, and perhaps other sites.
■ Teaching: Look for a general statement about teaching medical students or residents, unless you are being

recruited chiefly as an educator. In that case, the job description may describe more specific teaching duties.

- Scholarship: Scholarly expectations may be described generally. If this is a research position, look for a more complete discussion of duties.
- Administration: There may be mention of administrative duties, such as serving as head of a specialized clinic or becoming director of a continuing medical education program. If the job has no administrative role, the job description may be silent in this category.

Supervision/Reporting

This important statement tells whom you will report to directly. Ultimately, all faculty are responsible to the department chair and, thence, to the dean of the school. Your direct supervisor becomes important because that person determines much of what you do day by day and will also probably write your annual faculty evaluation.

Other Expectations

At the end of the position description, there might be a statement about the person filling the position being expected to act in an ethical manner and in accord with the mission of the institution. The absence of such a statement has no significance.

Requirements for the Position

Listed here will be some specific skills that applicants must bring to the job. Examples might be "five years experience working in an intensive care unit," "commitment to provide obstetrical care," "PhD or Doctor of Public Health degree," or "Certificate of Added Qualifications in Geriatrics."

What Is Negotiable in the Academic Job Description?

Some elements described above are negotiable, although you and I must recognize that the position description is a legal document, and the language protects both parties.

Position Title

The basic position title isn't likely to be negotiable, but it may be possible to add another duty. For example, you might expand "Clinician-Educator" to add "and Director of the Travel Medicine Clinic."

Requirements for the Position

Because of the legal risk to the institution of litigation from unsuccessful applicants, these requirements may not be negotiable.

Salary Range

Within the stated range, salary is definitely negotiable. Start your negotiation with the high end of the range, especially if your qualifications exceed the minimum "Requirements for the Position."

Full-Time Equivalent

This may be open to discussion. If the position offered is less than full-time, bargain hard to get to a level that brings fringe benefits.

Dates

The starting date is almost always negotiable.

Responsibilities

Be especially sure that you and the department chair (or whoever is negotiating for the chair) reach full agreement about your clinical responsibilities. This will very likely be spelled out in more detail in your Offer Letter (see Chapter 4).

Supervisor/Reporting

It is always best, if possible, to report directly to the top person. If this is not feasible, try to be sure that your supervisor reports directly to the chair. Seek to avoid two levels between you and the chair.

Other Expectations

The position description may indicate that you will be asked later to sign an "ethics" or "mission" statement, a document that is usually simply signed and filed. Interestingly, however, if the institution later claims that there is a problem with something you have done or are alleged to have done, the benign statement may become significant. Nevertheless, it is almost always pointless to attempt to negotiate a wording change in this statement when discussing a job.

FACULTY TRACKS AND RANKS

As we begin to consider faculty tracks and ranks, we bump head-on into the elitism than can occur in academic medical centers. Faculty tracks describe a type of appointment, and there are several ways of describing tracks. Faculty rank is a title that tells where you are in the academic pecking order.

Faculty Tracks

Faculty tracks can be a little confusing because of the diversity of expressions in various academic institutions. I find it useful to think of tracks as a dichotomous choice. The traditional tracks are *academic* (also often called *research*) versus *clinical*. The track is typically designated in the job description (see above).

Academic Track

This track connotes research, scholarship, and publications. This is the career pathway most of us think about when we think of academic medicine. Because those in the academic track bring in grant dollars, are actively involved in professional organizations, and otherwise enhance the reputation of the institution, academic/research faculty members are the favored sons and daughters of the dean, provost, and president.

Also, as we will see below, the publications, grant awards, and national offices that an individual accumulates on his or her curriculum vitae (CV) allow one to climb the promotion and tenure ladder. The academic track is sometimes called the *tenure track*, but this is not always precisely true, as explained below.

Without a few publications or grant awards on your CV, or at least some hint of future scholarly achievement, you are unlikely to receive an initial appointment to the academic track. Furthermore, you will find later that it is difficult to move from the clinical to the academic track, but it can be done.

Clinical Track

The recent residency/fellowship graduate or the practicing clinician entering academic medicine will probably be appointed to the clinical track. Three fourths of all allopathic medical schools have such a track.[1]

Medical schools may call these clinical tracks by various names. About half of the schools with clinical tracks characterize them and those in them as *clinical* or *clinician-educators*. Other terms you may encounter are *clinician-teachers*, *clinical pathway*, *clinical science*, or *clinical service*.[2]

Most clinical tracks require some sort of scholarship for advancement. In the clinical track, however, there is likely to be a somewhat liberal definition of scholarship. For example, a researcher on the academic track is expected to publish reports of original research in peer-reviewed journals. The faculty member on the clinical track can meet the requirements for scholarship in various ways. These include publishing review articles, case reports, and book chapters. Other scholarly options might be development of curricular or evaluation materials or creation of quality-assurance documents.[2] In my opinion, the lesser expectation for scholarly productivity in the clinical track is the chief reason for its diminished prestige.

Promotion is available to those in the clinical track, although one's rank may have a descriptive adjective appended to the designation of faculty rank (e.g., clinical assistant professor of surgery). Typically, individuals in clinical track are not eligible for tenure. This is true in at least 75% of U.S. medical schools.[2]

Tenure

That the concept of tenure exists in academic medicine represents the triumph of tradition over logic. Tenure originated in nonmedical academic institutions as a way to assure faculty the freedom to challenge dogma and follow unpopular paths of inquiry without fear of administrative or ideologic pressure. In short, a professor of English literature could not be fired for writing that Shakespeare was really a plagiarist. Nor could a physics professor be dismissed capriciously when a new chair was selected to head his or her department.

One difficulty of the tenure system has always been that once tenure is granted an individual, there is the tendency to "retire-in-place," and the institution finds that productivity by that professor dwindles. Furthermore, the presence of tenured senior faculty strolling into the sunset with full pay keeps talented junior faculty from advancing.

Today, research track academicians and, in a few academic medical centers, clinician-educators are eligible for, and earnestly seek, tenure. However, an institution and an individual academician may have decidedly different opinions about what tenure means. Clearly, with increasing pressures on institutional budgets, academic medical centers are seeking ways "to limit financial guarantees provided to clinical faculty members who are awarded tenure."[3] Some schools are modifying their tenure policy in a way that I believe will be the case in most medical schools that retain the tenure system in the future. The new model involves the legal stance that those who receive tenure are entitled to hold their academic positions until they retire. Holding the rank of tenured professor of internal medicine [or choose your specialty] does not, however, entitle one to receive a salary. Nor does it actually entitle one to an office, a desk, or a telephone. In reality, tenure under the evolving model only entitles one to write grants or see patients to support one's salary.

Another way in which institutions limit their tenure exposure is the time-limited award. For example, I might be awarded tenure for 5 years, with subsequent renewal dependent on a post-tenure review at the end of that time.

Schools that have not figured out what to do about tenure and tracks have developed "various employment and pay arrangements that inform or confuse the question."[3] The reality is that you should not count on institutional tenure to protect your job. Your true tenure is your clinical skills. If all fails in your academic career tomorrow, you should be able to open a practice in the community and earn a living. Clinicians, this—not a tenure award—is your job security.

Other Faculty Track Variations

As mentioned above, you will hear about *tenure* versus the *nontenure* tracks, the latter sometimes called *fixed-term* or *contract-term* appointments. To use my institution as an example, Oregon Health & Science University (OHSU) has no formal clinical track. We do, however, have fixed-term and tenure track appointments. Our statement of *Policies, Procedures and General Guidelines for Promotion and Tenure* states that, "It is implicit in the designation 'fixed-term appointment' that funding of a position cannot be guaranteed beyond a certain time period. Therefore, fixed-term appointment notices should clearly state that conversion from fixed-term to tenure track is not an automatic right."[4]

Faculty Ranks

Faculty ranks are a little less confusing than tracks and tenure. Fundamentally, whether you are in a clinical or academic track, there are four basic faculty ranks: instructor, assistant professor, associate professor, and professor. For each rank, there are requirements, but because they must apply to a wide variety of academic faculty members, the criteria are necessarily imprecise and are subject to interpretation. You must, in the typical institution, have evidence of contributions in the areas of teaching, scholarship, and service, the latter a broad category that includes clinical care.

Associate and full professor are considered senior faculty ranks. For promotion to the rank of associate professor, one should have achieved regional or national recognition for achievements. For professor, the bar raises to national or international recognition. A few academic institutions, such as the University of California system, also have gradations within ranks. An AMC may specifically lower the bar to regional recognition for senior faculty rank for those in a clinical track.

Some schools require that faculty be considered for promotion in rank or for tenure after a certain time—often 7 years. In many institutions that have such a rule, failure to be promoted or achieve tenure is not the end of your academic career. You may be permitted to continue working on a "fixed-contract" basis and be considered for promotion or tenure at a later time. When applying for an academic position, I recommend that you ask if there is an "up-or-out" promotion and tenure policy, and if the answer is yes, obtain a copy of the specific wording of the regulation.

I will discuss more about the promotion process in Chapter 3.

ACADEMIC COMPENSATION: GETTING PAID FOR WHAT YOU DO

Academic Medicine versus Private Practice Pay

Asking if you will earn more in academic medicine or private practice is a good place to start. Unfortunately, the answer is not clear because of many variables: these include your specialty, geographic location, and the inevitable interinstitutional differences. Portland, Oregon, for instance, is considered a desirable place to live, and this tends to be reflected in salary offers to new faculty at my institution.

For some generalities, let's look at interspecialty differences. Academic medical centers reflect the medical marketplace in that they "typically reward scarcity, so it shouldn't be surprising that some of the nation's most sought after specialists are significantly ahead in the earnings race."[5] In a Medical Economics (ME) survey of U.S physicians, the highest earners were invasive cardiologists, earning $360,000 per year.[5] Obstetrician/gynecologists earned an annual income of $220,000; family physicians and internists tied with incomes of $150,000; and pediatricians trailed with annual earnings of $116,000. The ME survey made no comparison of private practice with academic practice.

Hospitalists are a relatively new category, earning total compensation of $155,000 in a survey reported in 2004.[6] Again, the survey has no comparison of academic versus private practice salaries.

One thing we do know is that academic clinicians seem to generate less patient care income than their colleagues in private practice. In a study of 35 academic pediatricians, more than half of the faculty had clinical productivity that fell below the Medical Group Management Association (MGMA) 25th percentile.[7]

A MGMA 2003 report (based on 2002 data) reported salaries for some academic specialties. For that year, the median salary for a primary care faculty member was $132,000. Anesthesiologists earned $217,000; OB/GYNs $166,000; ophthalmologists $205,000; and infectious disease specialists $130,000. The highest paid academic specialists were cardiovascular surgeons, with an average total compensation of $368,000.[8]

If you are keenly interested in learning about average faculty salaries for filled, full-time faculty positions at U.S. medical schools, there is a summary available. The document is the American Association of Medical Colleges (AAMC) Annual Report on Medical School Faculty Salaries, available for sale from the AAMC in Washington, DC. However, seeing the AAMC tables does not provide a compelling advantage for the typical job applicant coming from residency, fellowship, or private practice. Salary tables are averages and are always outdated. A better comparison is to look at salary offers from various jobs available at the time you are applying for a position—not what was true 18–24 months ago.

Also, total salary comparisons with private practice and among academic institutions cannot account for the intangibles—fringe benefits, facilities provided by the institution, and potential for outside income—available to the academic clinician.

Academic Salaries: X, Y, and Z

Academic salaries are often described in terms of X, Y, and Z, often expressed as fractions of FTE. Here is what the letters represent:

- ■ X is the base salary. This amount may be an allocation from the departmental budget. Your clinical income and any grant awards may also be used to support part or all of your base salary.
- ■ Y is salary related to programmatic duties. The Residency Director will have a Y salary component. So might the Clinic Director, Director of Predoctoral (student) Education, and perhaps even the Director of Quality Assurance.
- ■ Z is practice-generated income.

Your total salary is the sum of the three (or perhaps two, if you have no programmatic duties with a salary attached, and hence no Y income).

One or Two Checks

Your salary may come to you in one or two checks, depending on the rules at your institution. Why might this be important? Your institutional check is likely to determine your level of fringe benefits, including payments into a faculty retirement account; federal, state, and local income taxes will be withheld. A second check from a faculty practice plan may or may not allow payments into a retirement account; income taxes may not be withheld and, if these payments are not deducted, you must allow for this in your personal tax accounting.

Faculty Practice Plans

In most institutions, clinicians will be both faculty members and participants in a faculty practice plan. The faculty practice plan describes a more-or-less private practice group that is related in some way to the institution but is governed by the clinicians. The practice group will have its own bank accounts and often its own retirement plan for clinicians. A governing board of practicing clinicians will make policy decisions, and there will probably be an executive director and several paid employees. In many institutions, the faculty practice plan is a very powerful player, with both organizational and financial clout.

Outside Income

One of the very nice benefits of academic practice is the opportunity to earn outside income. Possibilities include moonlighting, expert testimony, consulting honoraria, and royalties. In most institutions, outside income is yours to keep. A few parsimonious academic department chairs or deans claim one or more types of outside income as theirs.

Moonlighting

This may be the most problematic of the outside income possibilities. Your academic medical center or faculty practice group may prohibit off-campus work. If outside clinical work is prohibited, skip to the next heading. If allowed, you may choose to spend evenings and weekends working on contract for practices or hospitals in your community. The income from such work may come to you directly or might flow to you through the faculty practice group account.

A major consideration when considering outside clinical work is professional liability insurance. Be very certain that you are covered, whether through the your medical center, the institution hiring you, or your own policy.

Expert Testimony in Professional Liability Cases

After a few years on faculty, you are likely to receive the first of many telephone calls from the offices of attorneys. The question will be, "Would you like to review the records on a professional liability claim?" Your faculty status makes you a very credible expert in your field, and many academic faculty provide expert opinions in malpractice cases.

Be careful that you are not going to be testifying as an expert witness for one attorney and find yourself disagreeing with a faculty colleague who has been recruited by the adversary. Our institution seeks to avoid this by requesting that physicians who agree to testify as expert witnesses inform the university's legal office, which can help to avoid embarrassing conflicts in the courtroom.

The fees for being an expert witness can be substantial. A reasonable fee for young faculty serving in an expert witness role might be $300 per hour for record review and research, plus $3000 per day for testimony and travel. These fees are considered a replacement of what I could earn as gross income during the same time seeing patients, which is an important distinction if asked on the witness stand if you are being "paid for your testimony." Whatever you charge, in most settings, the fees are yours to keep.

Consulting Honoraria

Honoraria can come from many sources. A nearby company was developing a unique type of electrocardiograph and wanted an opinion about acceptability by primary care physicians; I greatly enjoyed learning about the innovative product and was happy to receive an honorarium for my opinion.

Some advertiser-sponsored medical publications pay $300 to $1000 to write review articles on clinical topics of interest to their readers. Such review articles are a logical early writing effort for young academicians.[9]

Royalties

Some academic clinicians write books and, as with article honoraria, these payments are generally yours to keep. Compiling a book is a major project; it should follow a history of writing review articles and perhaps some reports of clinical research.[9]

There also may be royalties attached to a clinical invention, such as a new device to deliver intravenous products. Academic medical centers typically distinguish between the written word and inventions as intellectual property. Hence the vagaries of institutional rules are likely to allow you to keep article and book royalties and consider inventions the property of the university.

GENDER DIFFERENCES IN ACADEMIC CAREERS

The special issues of women physicians have been an important topic for some time and have generated an increasing body of literature. For example, the book *Women in Medicine* by Bowman, Frank, and Allen is in its third edition.[10] More recent work concerns specific issues of women as faculty in academic medical centers—issues such as hiring, productivity, and career advancement, as well as isolation and gender discrimination.

Anyone who has been in a medical school classroom can attest to the fact that the gender composition of medical student bodies has changed radically over the past generation. When I was in medical school, about 7% of my class were women, and this was considered enlightened and progressive. Today, more than half of those in the first-year class at my medical school are women—some are married with children. On a national basis, 2003 was a pivotal year in which, for the first time in history, women were the majority of U.S. medical school applicants.[11]

Yet, the faculty at medical schools today are chiefly men, and senior faculty are especially likely to be male. In my opinion, the chief reason for the student versus faculty gender disparity is history. Faculty, and notably associate and full professors, began their careers 10–30 years ago, maybe more. And at that time, men predominated in medical schools and residencies. Thus, eventually, current trends seem likely to correct today's faculty gender disparities.

Other issues that challenge women in academia are an increased likelihood to work part-time and to avoid after-hours obligations, especially while their children are young. Also while raising young children, women might take a career hiatus, followed by the inevitably painful reentry and an effort to catch up.

Some Problems Studied

Career Experiences

Schroen and colleagues conducted a survey of 317 female and male members of the American College of Surgeons.[12]

Of the respondents, there were 168 men and 149 women. The researchers found gender differences in academic rank, tenure status, career aspirations, and income. In the sample studied, male surgeons had published a median of 25 articles compared with 10 articles for the women (P < 0.001). The authors concluded that being married or a parent did not influence the number of publications for the women.

In the study, overall career satisfaction was reported as high, but women were more likely than men to report feeling isolated from their surgical colleagues. The women surgeons reported feeling that career advancement opportunities were less available to them when compared with male surgeons. Of all respondents, 10–20% reported that they were considering leaving academia, and the individuals most likely to be considering this option were women assistant professors of surgery (29%).[12]

Career Advancement and Well-being

Researchers at Stanford University School of Medicine examined issues related to career success and the well-being of women faculty. In a survey of 163 women faculty in the medical school, respondents reported on the "climate" at the school and what they believed women needed to achieve their academic potential.[13]

Respondents reported that, compared with previous surveys conducted 7 and 8 years earlier, there had been a "nonsignificant decrease in mean ratings for sexual harassment, gender discrimination, and gender insensitivity in the intervening years." Over this same time interval, mean ratings for "climate and cohesion" remained stable.

The other half of the Stanford survey concerned needs. The 163 women academic faculty respondents identified the following needs, with mean rankings on a 5-point scale:

- Flexible work environment without negative consequences for women with young children (4.37)
- Three-month sabbatical from clinical and administrative duties (4.15)
- Departmental mentoring for academic career development (4.13)

■ School/departmental administrative secretarial support for grant and manuscript preparation (4.11)

Discrimination

Carr and colleagues examined gender discrimination in 18 women in academic medicine "who experienced or may have experienced discrimination in the course of their professional academic medical careers."[14] These women, from 13 different institutions, participated in interviews that covered the role of discrimination in hindering careers, coping mechanisms, and how the professional climate for women could be improved. Of the subjects, 40% "ranked gender discrimination first out of 11 possible choices for hindering their career in academic medicine." Another 35% ranked "limited time for professional work" or "lack of mentoring" as the leading career hindrance, with "gender discrimination" ranked second. The lack of women at high levels of the academic hierarchy was seen as a problem.

The authors conclude that, "According to this subset of women who perceive that they have been discriminated against based on gender, sexual bias and discrimination are subtly pervasive and powerful."

Gender Differences and Academia of the Future

Two decades ago, one of my good friends, now deceased, was one of the pioneer women chairs of a clinical department in a medical school. We served together on several national committees. In this setting she would grumble, "We discuss an important issue for an hour. Then we call a break and the men go into the restroom and make the decision."

I don't think this happens any more, at least not often. The trend toward equal gender numbers of men and women in academia will be a big help in solving the problem. If women come to outnumber men in medicine, as they do in some countries today, then in some future edition of this book, I might be writing about gender bias against men. It could happen.

ETHNIC/RACIAL DIFFERENCES IN ACADEMIC CAREERS

The outlook may not be as favorable when we examine ethnic/racial issues in academic careers. Although a study of physician graduates of Jefferson Medical College showed that "African American respondents were comparable with White respondents as to their medical careers, professional activities, and achievements," examination of academia seems to present a different picture. In the Jefferson study, "African Americans reported greater dissatisfaction than Whites with interactions with medical school faculty and administrators and with the medical school social environment."[15]

A study of 1979 full-time AMC faculty showed that, "Many minority faculty report experiencing racial/ethnic bias in academic medicine and have lower career satisfaction than other faculty. Despite this, minority faculty who reported experiencing racial/ethnic discrimination achieved academic productivity similar to that of other faculty."[16] In another study of an impressive 50,145 full-time U.S. medical school faculty, Fang and colleagues found that, "Our data indicate that minority faculty are promoted at lower rates compared with white faculty."[17]

The Future

Although women seem destined to achieve parity with men in academia over the next few decades, minority physicians cannot make a similar projection. Currently, underrepresented minorities account for only about 4% of full-time academic faculty at U.S. medical schools.[18] An increase in this low percentage would require an increase in minority students graduating from medical school, but this is not happening.

Today, 12.1% of Americans are self-identified as African American/Black; 0.9% are Native American; and 12% are Hispanic/Latino. These three minority groups thus account for approximately 25% of the U.S. population.[19] On the other hand, "over the past decade only 10% of medical school graduates were from underrepresented minority groups, despite initiatives such as the Association of American Medical Colleges' *Project 3000 by 2000*."[20]

From Despair May Come Hope

Although the figures cited above are distressing, they offer hope to the minority clinician seeking an academic position. If this describes you, you are considered a valuable candidate. You are likely to be courted earnestly and to receive one or more attractive employment offers. If you take the attitude that, "The trend changes with me," then you can make a difference during your career as an academic clinician.

SURPRISES ENCOUNTERED BY ACADEMIC CLINICIANS

At the beginning of this chapter, I stated that I would begin and end with subjective data—the feelings and opinions of academic clinicians. Earlier I told what academicians like and don't like about their jobs. Here I will describe some surprises that the contributors and I have encountered.

I have grouped the surprises into two categories: my personal surprises and those reported by contributors. Certainly, medical academics has changed—at least in some ways—since my entry in 1978. For this reason, we would expect my personal, early career surprises to be somewhat different from those reported currently by contributors. Are they? I leave it for you to decide.

Dr. Taylor's Surprises When Entering Academic Medicine

I entered academic medicine from solo, rural practice. In private practice, I not only needed to be a good doctor, but I also had to administer a practice; this meant getting office space, hiring a staff, developing a record system, setting up a billing method, creating an appointment scheme, and much more. I was in practice alone, and lack of attention to any of these items could cause chaos in the office and financial problems for my family. I tell you this because I believe that coming from a self-sustaining private practice made me keenly aware of how different academic medicine is. I encountered much that I had not anticipated.

Paying Your Way

In Chapter 1, I describe how academic departments—and the faculty in these departments—have a "hunting license" rather than a firm budget from the institution. Some medical schools allocate each department a "base budget" that is chiefly intended to support medical student and resident teaching plus some administrative services. Not all departments have even a small base budget and must look to other sources for salary and programmatic support.

Although you may not realize it at the time of being hired, you must earn your salary in some way. Patient care is the usual way, especially for new clinical faculty. The other major source of funds is grants, chiefly research grants. (I will tell more about grants and how to get them in Chapter 6.) Most medical schools and clinical departments receive little operating income from gifts and endowments.

What this means is this: The department chair must patch together your salary support every year, and you must help. If you slack off on patient care or spend too much time away at meetings, you are likely to see your income drop. If you depend on grant support for a chunk of your income and you fail to get an important grant one year, your department may give you some "tiding over" money for a short time. Eventually, you must get your grant, see more patients, or cut back on your FTE time.

Teaching Is Undervalued

Imagine my surprise to learn that teaching is not highly appreciated by colleagues. The devaluation of teaching is ironic, as education is what defines a medical school, and without a medical school there is no AMC. Once, after a few years in academics, I was offered the opportunity to lead our department's predoctoral education program—to be in charge of our faculty's medical school teaching efforts. A senior faculty member called me aside and counseled me not to take the job. His reason, "Teaching is a dead-end path. You will never get promoted."

As a matter of fact, I now believe that working with medical student programs is an excellent career pathway to becoming a department chair or dean. After all, chairman and dean positions are in the *medical school* arena. Nevertheless, the antiteaching bias continues to exist.

I recommend an article in JAMA by DeAngelis titled "Professors Not Professing."[21] The message is profound and I am going to quote the author:

> "The title most sought by academicians is 'professor.' Ironically, it is most difficult to achieve this goal as a medical educator. In fact, in most medical schools, the more time a faculty member spends teaching, the less likely she or he would become a professor, especially a 'professor' with no adjective attached."

The author goes on to cite a JAMA article showing that, in a sample of more than 100,000 academicians, 35.5% of basic science faculty (who are primarily researchers) are professors compared with 21.1% of clinical faculty (who are likely to spend as much or more time teaching as do the basic science faculty).[11]

The Physicians Are Not in Charge
In private practice, I could control my work hours, appointment templates, and fee schedule; in academic medicine, administrators are likely to define the context of your patient care. Most academic medical centers are top-heavy with administrators. This includes an army of hospital and clinic managers who spend their time trying to regulate the lives of clinicians. Sudden announcements of policy changes in the hospital and clinics are the norm. New forms and other paperwork burdens seem to be introduced daily. One day I received an e-mail from clinics administration stating that on a certain prenatal visit encounter form, if I did not initial one small box on the form, I would not be paid for the care. I doubt that any practicing clinician participated in this decision.

The Physicians Are Not Always Highly Respected
In the academic setting, nurses and physicians sometimes have more testy relationships than in private practice settings. My residents report much different interactions with

nurses and staff during community hospital rotations than they find in the teaching hospital. I think that the teaching hospital nurses have spent a great deal of time working with struggling learners and have lost the respect for physicians that is more common in the private setting.

Opportunities Abound

When I entered academics, I anticipated that my life would become richer and more diverse than in solo, country practice. But I had no idea. My granddaughter has a disco ball, also called a mirror ball. You have seen them, reflecting light on small mirrors, creating a scintillating image that is almost disorienting. This is the way I—like many freshly minted academicians—found the new job to be.

For example, in a given morning, I might attend a breakfast meeting, see some patients with residents, answer e-mails, discuss a research project with colleagues, talk with some residents in the hallway, dictate a letter, and return telephone calls—all before lunch.

Today, as a senior faculty member, I receive invitations to speak here and abroad, and I am chairing an international meeting next month. I help young faculty with their scholarly projects, lead our department's fund-raising, teach medical students in small-group seminars, and serve as attending physician for residents in their clinical care. I also write and edit books for clinicians.

For those of us who enjoy a variety of challenges and like keeping busy, this is wonderful. For the person who likes to focus on a single topic, to do one thing and do it very well, over and over, academics can be overwhelming.

Being Entrepreneurial Is the Key to Success

Who would guess it? The most successful academic clinicians are the entrepreneurs—the go-getters who can find a need and fill it with a flair. Whether it is a breast service, a cochlear implant center, or an integrative medicine clinic, the academic medical center rewards narrow specialization and an innovative spirit.

What does this mean for the generalist? Is there no hope for the general internist or family physician? Yes, there are entrepreneurial opportunities available for generalists. In family medicine and general internal medicine, we have special clinics for sports medicine, geriatrics, pain management, weight control, headache management, and more. The key for the generalist is to look beyond specialty boundaries, and find an area—often a symptom such as "headache" or "pain" rather than, let's say, hypertension—that is turf not already dominated by a single specialty.

Contributors' Surprises

I asked contributors, "What have been the pleasant and the unpleasant surprises about being an academic clinician?" What follows is a "brain-stormed" list, with happy and unhappy comments presented in random order (and editorial comments in italic):

- "There aren't enough hours to do everything I want to do."
- "I am continually impressed with the quality of our medical students and residents. They are so outstanding that I sometimes wonder if I would be accepted to medical school today."
- "A pleasant surprise has been the wonderfully collaborative spirit of my colleagues."
- "I think that one of the best parts of my day is having lunch with colleagues. We discuss some of the medical issues of the day, and it is as good as any CME program around."
- "A pleasant surprise? The appreciation of those we teach."
- "The residents aren't interested in my experience. For clinical decisions, they want to know the evidence in the literature." (*We all soon learn that learners have little interest in "war stories."*)
- "My job let me build my computer skills in a way I could never do on my own. And there is always a technician available if I have a problem with my hardware."
- "Today's students and residents don't seem to be willing to work as hard as we did in our time."

- "I have so many thing to do and so many people asking me to do more, that I feel like I am being pecked to death by chickens."
- "It doesn't take very long for your students to come back and say that you've been an important influence in their lives."
- "I'm never bored."
- "An unpleasant surprise has been the remuneration in comparison to private practice."
- "Life is more predictable."
- "A big surprise has been the marginal funding of teaching programs and faculty positions in most schools."
- "I don't have the administrative support I need. I share a secretary with three other faculty members. This means that I do most of my own document preparation, photocopying, and appointment scheduling."
- "I find that I am willing to forgo clinical activities for those that are intellectually stimulating, but not directly remunerative."
- "I never realized how much teaching and administration is done by PhD and master's degree faculty. Our academic department couldn't get along without them, and neither could I when I am doing research or writing a paper."
- "You have to wear many hats, and each of these roles can fill an entire career."
- "The quality of care in the academic medical center is not as high as I expected. The really good, young doctors go into private practice."
- "It has been eye-opening how much fun it is, and how hard the work is. I remember as a resident, a senior academician in our specialty came to our program and stated that academic work was harder than full-time practice. I was skeptical. He was right. But it is more fun and rewarding, at least for me, and I enjoyed community practice very much."
- "The declining financial support for higher education in our state."
- "There is little opportunity to do research. I seem to spend all my time seeing patients and doing chart work."
- "Paperwork."

- "You need to check everything with everybody. Any time I have a good idea, I need to get approval from ten different people. There is so much bureaucratic red tape here that you can't get anything done."
- "I really enjoy the time I get to spend on research."
- "Many people in the medical school environment lack the kind of professionalism and idealism I expect from teachers."
- Before I entered academics, I used to say, "I hate meetings." The surprise is that I have come to realize that meetings are how you move things ahead around here. I hate to admit it, but I am getting to enjoy meetings."
- "I find that the better job you do, the more work people tend to give you."
- "I need to be very careful about stepping on other people's toes. Last year I got a small grant to provide some free medication to diabetic patients among our seasonal farm worker population. Sounds like a good idea, right? I then found I had caused a problem and that I was in trouble. Why? Because someone in another department had a big grant proposal having to do with diabetic farm workers that she had planned to submit to the same agency. We got there first, and she 'lost' a major grant opportunity."
- Because I have a supportive chair, I've been able to pursue educational interests and develop expertise in technology and its use in education."
- "If I had known that academic medicine was so much fun, I would have looked for a teaching job right out of residency."
- "I've been successful in academic medicine, not because I've aspired to be successful, but simply by doing the best job I can day by day, and taking advantage of opportunities that arise."
- "Unpleasant surprises? None so far." (*This comment is from a relatively new faculty member.*)

There seems to be a balance of pleasant and unpleasant surprises about academic careers. To learn more, let us go on to Chapter 3 in which I discuss the academic medical center.

REFERENCES

1. Jones RF, Gold JS. Faculty appointment and tenure policies in medical schools. Acad Med 1998;73:211–219.
2. Society of Academic Emergency Medicine: Faculty Development Website. Available at http://www.saem.org/facdev/mainpages/clinical_track.htm/.
3. Jones RF, Gold JS. The present and future of appointment, tenure, and compensation policies for medical school clinical faculty. Acad Med 2001;76:993–1004.
4. Oregon Health & Science University School of Medicine. Policies, procedures and general guidelines for promotion and tenure. November 2, 2000. Portland, OR: OHSU.
5. Guglielmo WJ. Physicians' earnings. Medical Economics. Available at http://www.memeg.com/.
6. Hospitalists are earning a healthy living. Med Econ 2004; July 9: p. 18.
7. Andreae MC, Freed GL. Using a productivity-based physician compensation program at an academic health center: a case study. Acad Med 2002;77:894–899.
8. Physicians Money Digest. 2003; Aug. 31: p. 21.
9. Taylor RB. The clinician's guide to medical writing. New York: Springer-Verlag, 2005.
10. Bowman MJ, Frank E, Allen DI. Women in medicine, 3rd ed. New York: Springer-Verlag, 2002.
11. Barzansky B, Etzel SI. Educational programs in US medical schools, 2003–2004. JAMA 2004;292:1025–1031.
12. Schroen AT, Brownstein MR, Sheldon GF. Women in academic surgery. Acad Med 2004;79:310–318.
13. McGuire LK, Bergen MR, Polan ML. Career advancement for women faculty in a U.S. school of medicine: perceived needs. Acad Med 2004;79:319–325.
14. Carr PL, Szalacha L, Barnett R, Caswell C, Inui T. A "ton of feathers": gender discrimination in academic medical careers and how to manage it. J Womens Health 2003;12:1009–1018.
15. Gartland JJ, Hojat M, Christian EB, Callahan CA, Nasca TJ. African American and white physicians: a comparison of satisfaction with medical education, professional careers, and research activities. Teach Learn Med 2003;15(2):106–112.
16. Peterson NB, Friedman RH, Ash AS, Franco S, Carr PL. Faculty self-reported experience with racial and ethnic discrimination in academic medicine. J Gen Intern Med 2004; 19:259–265.

17. Fang D, Moy E, Colburn L, Hurley J. Racial and ethnic disparities in faculty promotion in academic medicine. JAMA 2000;284:1085–1092.

18. Erwin DO, Henry-Tillman RS, Thomas BR. A qualitative study of the experiences of one group of African Americans in pursuit of a career in academic medicine. J Natl Med Assoc 2002;94: 802–812.

19. US Census Bureau. Data for 2000 Census: Available at http://www.census.gov/population/www/cen2000/briefs.html/.

20. Lypson ML, Gruppen L, Stern DT. Warning signs of declining faculty diversity. Acad Med 2002;77:S10–S12.

21. DeAngelis CD. Professors not professing. JAMA 2004;292: 1060–1061.

3

What You Need to Know About the Academic Medical Center

In the past chapter, I discussed an academic career and what it can mean for you as a clinician. In this chapter, I will tell about the academic medical center (AMC)—where academic clinicians work. I will give an overview of the medical center's organizational structure, governance, and culture. I will also tell about its value and reward system, with a special emphasis on promotion and tenure. Near the end of the chapter you will find a valuable summary of "unwritten rules" of medical academia, as shared by our contributors; I find this list as fascinating as the answers are diverse.

THE ACADEMIC MEDICAL CENTER

America's academic medical centers are national treasures. This statement is no exaggeration. In the AMCs (sometimes called academic health centers) we find the resources for patients with the most rare and challenging diseases, research and scholarship that brings us the drugs and inventions that literally save lives, and education for tomorrow's physicians, scientists, and others in the health care field. Considered in the context of a sports metaphor, America's AMCs are like well-funded major league baseball teams capable of hiring the truly superstar players—clinicians and researchers.

Once AMCs were simply considered trade schools. They represented an industry that produced a product—future practitioners to serve America and other areas of the world. Today the AMC can be considered the poster child for the transition from an industrial to an information society.

Medical academicians sometimes grumble about pay, gripe about teaching loads, scheme to get coveted grants and space, and assail one another—at least one another's ideas. But in our hearts we know that we spend our days in an incredibly enriched and privileged setting, and most of us wouldn't work anywhere else. The best evidence is the many retired academic clinicians—like me—who continue to work in the AMC for little or no pay.

Exactly what is an academic medical center? In "About This Book," I provided an easy working definition: An academic medical center includes a medical school, a teaching hospital affiliation, and a research program. Federal law (the Stark rule) defines an "academic medical center" as consisting of:

■ An accredited medical school (including a university, when appropriate);
■ An affiliated faculty practice plan [*hint: the Stark law is about payment for patient care*];

and

■ One or more affiliated hospital(s) in which a majority of the hospital medical staff consists of physicians who are faculty members and a majority of all hospital admissions are made by physicians who are faculty members.[1]

To this "stark" definition, I would add that a medical center fulfills three vital functions: education, patient care, and scholarship. Without all three elements, the institution may be something else, but it is not an academic medical center. A single institution may actually govern all three enterprises, but there are exceptions: Harvard University runs no clinical practice and owns no hospitals; Harvard sends its students to various *affiliated* hospitals in the Boston area.[2]

Whenever using a word, I like to explore its origins; this exercise helps me to remember the word and—I hope—to use it correctly. "Academic" comes from *Academia*, the name of a grove in Athens, Greece. It was here that Plato taught his pupils.[3]

And the allusion to ancient Greece brings us to the origins of academic medical centers.

Origins of Academic Medical Centers

In terms of history, academic medical centers are very new. According to Asimov, the earliest example of *Homo sapiens* is Neanderthal man, which makes our species at least 100,000 years old.[4] Thinking of human history to date in terms of a 24-hour day, academic medical centers arise barely a second before midnight. In this short section, I will tell about three landmarks in the evolution of AMCs: the early days in Greece; the first centers in America; and the changes that followed the Flexner report.

Academic Medicine in Ancient Greece

I don't think anyone can say when and where the first AMC began, and so I am going to describe what must have been one of the oldest and certainly one of the most famous locations—the temple of Aesculapius on the Greek island of Cos.

Cos was, of course, the island home of Hippocrates (c. 460–377 BC), called by some the Father of Medicine and considered a direct descendent of Aesculapius[3] (see Figure 3.1). Aesculapius is the ancient Greek god of medicine; legend holds that he is the son of Apollo, the god of healing, and a mortal woman named Coronis. In fact, Aesculapius was probably a man who lived about 1200 BC. One of the best-known shrines to Aesculapius is at Cos in the Peloponnese.[3] I have special warmth for this place because, as a member of a physician tour group, I visited this site in 2002 and in unison we recited the oath of Hippocrates outdoors on a bright, sunny day (see Figures 3.2A and 3.2B).

I choose Cos as the early shining example because here Hippocrates and his colleagues fulfilled the three main functions of an AMC. They treated sick patients, they taught students, and they engaged in clinical inquiry—largely observational—and wrote about it as examples of scholarship that endure today.

Coming to America

AMCs evolved and matured through the centuries, chiefly in Europe and Asia. Eventually they found their way to the New World.

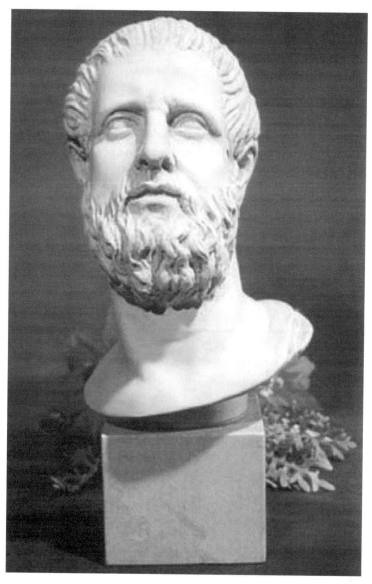

Figure 3.1. Hippocrates (c. 460–377 BC).

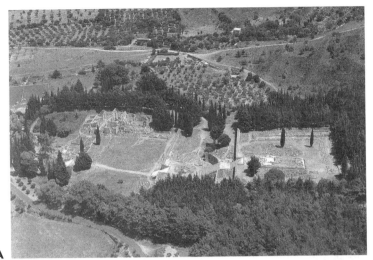

A

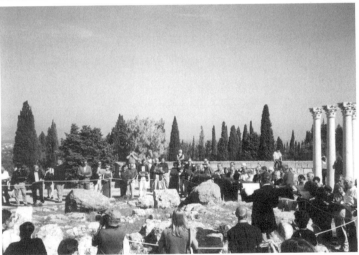

B

FIGURE 3.2. (A) The Temple of Aesculapius on the Island of Cos. (B) American physicians reciting the Oath of Hippocrates at the Shrine of Aesculapius on the Island of Cos.

Until the 1760s, none of the institutions of higher learning in the American colonies had a department of medicine. Medical education was largely based on an apprentice model, and the practitioners who mentored these apprentices might, in fact, have had no formal medical education.[5] The first academic medical center in the United States began with the establishment of the medical department of the College of Philadelphia in 1765. This department, affiliated with the Pennsylvania Hospital, was founded by Doctors John Morgan and William Shippen, Jr. Dr. Shippen was the author of *A Discourse upon the Institution of Medical Schools in America*. Morgan and Shippen thus combined education, patient care, and scholarship.[5]

In 1768, a medical department was added to King's College in New York City, but—amazing as it may seem—there was no hospital in New York at that time.[5]

The Flexner Report
In 1910, a landmark document changed American medical education forever. Abraham Flexner wrote: "If the sick are to reap the full benefit of recent progress in medicine, a more uniformly arduous and expensive medical education is demanded."[6] Flexner called for reforms in four areas:

■ Establishment of educational standards for medical schools
■ Emphasis on the scientific basis of medical education
■ Insistence on clinical teaching under close supervision in the setting of a teaching hospital under the control of the medical faculty
■ Development of a full-time faculty to teach clinical medicine[7]

In short, the Flexner report and the response of American medicine standardized medical education, started the rise of science—read *research*—in medicine, and ended the apprenticeship model of training future doctors.

There were, however, some unintended consequences of the Flexner report. Most small, medical colleges in rural towns were closed, resulting in physician shortages in many localities. Only two African-American medical colleges survived, with the resultant decrease in opportunities for medical training for minority young people. As medical education became not only more arduous but also expensive, a professional elitism arose. One casualty was primary care, as the Flexner reforms began a decline in generalism that was corrected only with the rise of family medicine beginning in 1969.[7-9]

TYPES OF ACADEMIC MEDICAL CENTERS

America has 126 medical schools accredited by the Liaison Committee on Medical Education. There are also 19 U.S. schools of osteopathic medicine accredited by the American Osteopathic Association. Canada has 17 medical schools. Lists of these schools are found in the Appendix.

The magazine *U.S. News and World Report* provides an annual ranking of both research and primary care medical schools.[10] Some medical schools are considered research oriented and receive major funding from National Institute of Health (NIH) research grants. Harvard, Washington University, and Johns Hopkins fall into this category. Other medical schools are best known for primary care education. The University of Washington in Seattle, the University of North Carolina at Chapel Hill, and Oregon Health & Science University topped the 2006 Primary Care list. Some schools, such as the University of Iowa College of Medicine, are "bimodal," highly successful in both obtaining research funding and producing primary care physicians.[11]

This ranking is based on a methodology that is considered flawed by many, especially by those medical schools not ranked highly on the lists; however, medical students and academicians alike pay attention to the rankings.

ACADEMIC MEDICAL CENTER GOVERNANCE

Medical center governance continues to baffle many, including those like me who have spent decades as academicians. It is a system that can cause a businessperson to gasp in confusion. How can such a complicated system function?

By all principles of aerodynamics, with its small, delicate wings relative to its body size, the hummingbird cannot fly. With its huge tail and almost vestigial legs, the alligator cannot run. And with the bizarre organizational structure shown in Figure 3.3, the academic medical center cannot function as an institution. (As I think about it, it is illogical that the *Tyrannosaurus rex* is extinct, and yet sheep, dim-witted and vulnerable, have survived until the 21st century.)

Of course, the hummingbird can fly, and an alligator in Florida was able to run—at least for a short distance—fast enough to catch and eat my nephew's dog. And somehow,

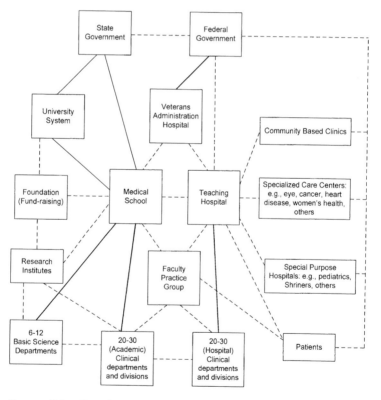

FIGURE 3.3. Organizational chart of an academic medical center. Solid lines indicate reporting relationships; dotted lines indicate affiliation relationships.

improbably, the academic medical center manages to govern itself, however sometimes inefficiently and often quite clumsily.

Figure 3.3 is a theoretical example of an academic medical center, and it is likely that no single institution exactly fits the model. For example, I have drawn the organizational chart to show a state-supported university system with a school of medicine, with solid lines (indicating reporting relationships) connecting the state government to the university system and the school of medicine. For a private institution—not state supported—these would probably be dotted lines (indicating affiliation relationships). Many academic medical centers include Veterans Administration hospitals, which provide student and resident teaching and which collaborate with the university hospital in providing various types of specialized patient care. The federal government has an ongoing relationship with university hospitals through its funding of graduate medical education. Each year the U.S. government, through its Medicare subsidy program, provides more than $5 billion in support of resident training.

The faculty practice group is generally a powerful force in the scheme. In Figure 3.3, I show no solid lines for this affiliated entity, indicating the autonomy the practice group usually enjoys. Although the medical school dean is sometimes the head of the practice group, such a role is likely to be one of consensus-builder, with the "real" power vested in the heavy-hitter clinical specialists, generally the high-profile surgeons. Of course, the person with the largest bank account at the AMC is likely to be the hospital director.

In order to avoid making the diagram even more complex, I omitted boxes for medical students and residents. Were I to add them, medical students would relate directly to the medical school, to whom they pay tuition. Residents would relate to the hospital, which pays their salary—with generous federal assistance.

Note the small box for "Patients" in the lower right-hand corner.

As you spend time in academia, you will come to realize that governance occurs in two ways: The first is through a formal, explicit system of authority; in business, we would call this a hierarchy, but Figure 3.3 shows why this word is inappropriate in an AMC. The second method by which governance occurs is the informal, unwritten system of personal relationships, networks, and trade-offs.

Professional School Departments and the Dean

The main power in the academic medical center is found in the professional departments, chiefly the clinical departments, because they control most of the available funding. Clinical departments are headed by department chairs, who hold considerable organizational power. The department chair can decide salaries, clinic assignments, and laboratory space allocations within his or her department. Chairs can hire and fire faculty, as long as they follow institutional guidelines. They generally enjoy a generous measure of budgetary autonomy. Clinical chairs are the last of the feudal lords.

The job of the dean is to govern the departments and maintain harmony among the feudal lords. My colleague, John Saultz, uses a metaphor from the science of physics: He holds that the powerful autonomy of the individual departments creates a *centrifugal force* that is not necessarily in the best interests of the school. The dean's task is to create a *centripetal force*, to bring the departments together to achieve the common mission(s) of the institution.

Institutional Finances

Most of the entities in Figure 3.3 have cash flow and reserve funds. This includes central administration, the medical school dean, the university hospital, clinical departments, the research institute, the Veterans Administration hospital, and the faculty practice group. The game is this: Each is busily trying to find ways to get money from the others. The dean will tax the income of practicing physicians to get money for education. The clinical departments will ask the Veterans Administration hospital to pay some or all of the salary support for clinicians who see their patients. The clinical departments ask the dean for salary support in return for teaching medical students. And so it goes.

Budgeting within a department is convoluted, necessitated by the many rules imposed by the federal government, funding agencies, private foundations, targeted grant awards, donor stipulations, and university rules. It is not uncommon for a clinical department to have 30 accounts or more, listed with the medical school, practice plan, and university foundation. The chief reason for the large number of accounts is the need to establish a new account for each research grant award received.

A current focus in AMCs is mission-based budgeting. This is an overt attempt, generally by an enlightened and courageous dean, to link departmental allocations of institutional dollars with teaching activity. In the future, allocations may even be based on outcomes (such as students choosing primary-care careers or rural practice or research fellowships) instead of on activities (such as teaching hours).[12] The alternative to mission-based budgeting is historical budgeting, in which departments receive more-or-less the educational budget they received last year and a decade ago. Whenever mission-based budgeting is undertaken, there is at first resistance and obfuscation in an attempt to retain historical budgeting. When implemented, mission-based budgeting is immediately followed by gamesmanship, with departments finding ways to inflate their educational effort reports. Mission-based budgeting, although a concept being actively pursued in many institutions, is still a work in progress.

Institutional Culture

Each academic medical center has its own culture, and within each AMC, each department has its own culture. Although I will not name institutions as examples (as I did with "research" and "primary care" medical schools above), it is clear that some schools have an intense, elitist, competitive culture, whereas other institutions have cultures that are collaborative, egalitarian, and benign. Within each school, individual departments may vary somewhat from the overall institutional culture, but not too much.

How can you tell about the culture before committing to work there? In interviews, you must ask pointedly, "Do faculty here work collaboratively or competitively?" "Can you tell me an example of cooperation between departments in grant-getting and research?" "Is there someone who has recently left the institution whom I could call to seek an opinion?"

Although medical schools are rarely in overall organizational distress owing to the diffusion of power, individual departments are sometimes unhappy and occasionally in chaos. In *Anna Karenina*, Tolstoy wrote, "Happy families are all alike; every unhappy family is unhappy in its own way." Troubled departments can have many causes: power struggles, warring factions, harassment of various types, impairment of the leader, financial failure of the clinical practice, and so forth. If you are considering joining a troubled department as a junior faculty member believing that you can fix the problems or that things can't get worse, I urge you to reconsider.

From time to time, a clinical department undergoes a cataclysm. Doom prevails and a major upheaval is underway. Faculty and staff are leaving as rapidly as possible. This situation is generally followed by the appointment of a new leader and perhaps an infusion of funds to get things back on track. Living through a cataclysm can be intensely painful, even damaging to the individual. Signing on to join a department rising from the ashes with a new leader can be a great opportunity—if the right leader has been chosen.

THE ACADEMIC MEDICAL CENTER VALUE SYSTEM

What is valued in the academic medical center? The answers may not be exactly what you think. I am going to go out on a limb and propose a hierarchy of what is valued. In descending order of importance, I believe that academic medical centers value: the creation of new knowledge;

clinical ability, especially a special skill; ability to get money; administrative abilities; teaching; and service to your colleagues, community, and specialty.

Creation of New Knowledge

Today's academic clinician must juggle clinical care, teaching, and scholarship. For those seeking academic career advancement—read *promotion* and perhaps *tenure*, *speaking invitations*, and *national recognition*—scholarly achievement is the key.

Without doubt, the scholarly imperative can be a burden for the academic clinician. As one who was in community practice for 14 years, I recall nostalgically the mental freedom afforded by attending solely to patient care: I had no educational curriculum to develop, no small groups to teach, no data to analyze, no papers to write. Yes, there was the occasional student from Albany Medical Center sent to have an experience in rural practice. Also, I did write a few papers for publication, but this is not typical of what practicing doctors do now. But, virtually all my professional energy centered on care of my patients and how to make that care better. In fact, my early articles were about just that—how to make your practice more efficient and provide better patient care.

Many in academics hold that the creation of new knowledge is the one distinctive role of the academician. This is probably true; one can see patients, raise money, administer organizations, teach, and serve in many other settings. Creating new knowledge is what AMCs do best. This means that if you list the reasons why you are considering a move to academic medicine and if scholarship is not somewhere on your list, you must ask if you are making the right career move.

One can write review papers, case reports, book chapters and even entire books, but the valued contribution is the "important" research paper published in a leading medical journal. Applegate and Williams write: "In general, young academicians should place greater emphasis on producing quality work than on generating a large quantity of work. A few high quality research publications in a focused field will further one's career and reputation as an 'expert' quite rapidly."[13]

The paragraph above can be discouraging to the new academic clinician, but I hope that will not be so. I present the "scholarly imperative" in academia and the value placed on high-quality work to persuade you to begin on day one to develop an area of scholarly interest, find a mentor with research experience, and join a research team to learn how to create new knowledge, whether in the clinical or educational arena.

Clinical Ability

The ability to provide outstanding patient care is highly valued in the AMC simply because, for the most part, we are describing a professional society of healers. From general pediatricians to cardiothoracic surgeons, superior medical knowledge and clinical skills are vitally important. Whatever your specialty, if you can practice it well you are likely to be respected by your colleagues. What does practicing your specialty well mean? It includes making solid and evidence-based clinical decisions, being attentive to your patients' needs, requesting timely and appropriate referrals, attending the necessary hospital meetings, and generally being a good professional colleague.

With that said, most highly valued is the clinician with a special skill. AMCs are, after all, the home of the sub-sub-specialist. There seem to be few broad-base clinicians here. Everyone has a favorite organ or disease: the thyroid, the retina, the knee, diabetes mellitus, prostate cancer, and so forth.

The exceptions are the true generalists: family physicians, general internists, and general pediatricians. In the academic setting, generalists begin at a disadvantage owing to their lack of a defining disease or procedure and to their somewhat lesser practice incomes. Some generalists respond by developing an "epispecialty"—an area of interest such as sports medicine, adolescent medicine, geriatrics, school health, alternative medicine, pain management, end-of-life care, and others. In a world of limited specialists, such focused expertise can prove useful in both practice and research.

Fund-raising

In academic medicine, whether generalist or subspecialist, the individual who can find funding will always have a job. In Chapter 1, I wrote of your salary designation really being a "hunting license." Well, the best hunters will always be welcome at the table.

Fund-raisers "hunt" in many areas. The traditional area is research grants, especially National Institutes of Health (NIH) grants. Some research grants are portable—they can move with you if you take a new job, giving you immense career flexibility. In the generalist specialties, there are Title 7 grants, which require special writing skills. Development work—soliciting donations from the community—is another valued activity, often helping to augment a department's or a medical school's revenues; someone other than a clinician generally does this sort of fund-raising, but not always.

If you want job security in academic medicine, find a way to fund your position.

Administrative Aptitude

The highest base salaries often go to those who administrate their departments and divisions. This is probably fair, because these individuals have stressful, high-burnout jobs; must function within the organizational milieux depicted in Figure 3.3; and have less time to earn patient-care income.

On the other hand, with administrative roles comes power—the ability to control the actions and even the careers of others. In the clinical department, the key administrative position is department chair. Others might include residency director, research director, clinic director, and hospital service director.

Seek an administrative role if you want to advance in the organizational hierarchy—and if you don't mind meetings, personnel issues, regulations, and paperwork.

Teaching

And finally we get to teaching.

Medical students value good teaching, but they do not sit on committees that determine who gets the rewards of academia (discussed below). Course directors also appreciate those who teach but have few perquisites to distribute. Until now, the system has not done a good job of rewarding the good teachers.

Perhaps things are changing. Mission-based budgeting can help reward those who teach. And the promotion system, long fossilized in tradition, is showing signs of reform. Hafler and Lovejoy report that, "The academic culture at Harvard Medical School has shifted from promotion based solely on original scholarship to promotion based on a broad array of educational contributions. The faculty, as they seek promotion, create portfolios that list written scholarship, teaching, and service at the local, regional, and national levels and at all ranks of promotion."[14]

Service

Service includes participating in committees, task forces, commissions, boards, and search committees. For young faculty, service can be a great way to network outside your department. I especially recommend that the new young faculty member volunteer to spend a year or two on the institutional review board that approves research protocols. Also included in service is time devoted to national professional organizations. Here you might seek a leadership role and join one of the many committees.

Community service is also valued. Volunteer for a local, county, or state task force if one is available. Work with a local charity. Join a service club. All these activities make you a better person and help advance the prestige of your AMC as being involved in the community.

THE ACADEMIC REWARD SYSTEM

Academicians are rewarded in various ways, and the method of allocating these rewards may seem as mysterious as most of the rest of what happens in AMCs. Some apparently worthy academic clinicians may receive low salaries, work harder than their colleagues, and suffer small, stuffy work quarters. Other academicians in the same department may fare much better. Who gets what benefits and why depends on the culture of the department, the pleasure of the chair, the longevity of the faculty member, and where that faculty member fits into the institutional power structure.

The many rewards include salary, of course; office space and equipment; access to administrative support; time for research and scholarship; teaching opportunities; travel time and allowance; and promotion and tenure. Salary is probably the lead consideration to most individuals, at least until they reach the transition into retirement. The others can be considered perquisites—a benefit above one's salary. Because different academic clinicians regard various of these nonmonetary rewards as more important than others, I have not listed them in any special order.

Salary

In Chapter 2, I discussed academic compensation, including the XYZ calculation, the one and two check systems, and how your salary is determined. If you are negotiating for a new position, keep in mind that your initial base salary— the X salary—is important, because subsequent raises are usually awarded as a percentage of this amount. For example, the dean may announce that, "This year all faculty will receive a pay increase amounting to 2 percent of base salary." The Y component of salary is a negotiation with your chair about special duties, such as serving as residency director. The Z part of your income is dependent on prac- tice revenue. If you want the Z figure to be greater, you just need to practice longer hours, bill a little higher, or see more patients in the time allotted.

Of course, little of this may apply to your situation. I know of several clinical departments in which the chair takes all the money, including base salary and practice income, and then tells each clinician how much he or she will receive next fiscal year.

Office Space and Equipment

Most academicians have two offices: their clinical area (often not an actual "office") and an academic office. Academic clinicians are likely to spend most of their time in patient care and thus in the clinical areas. For the neurosurgeon, this area is the operating room and surgical floors in the hospital. For the outpatient-oriented physician—endocrinologist, dermatologist, family physician, or psychiatrist—the chief practice setting will be an outpatient clinic of some type. Here there will be desirable exam rooms and inconvenient, cramped rooms. There will be helpful support staff and some who are frankly a little lazy. You will need to negotiate carefully to get the exam rooms and staff that can help make you most productive. This negotiation, however, generally is made after you accept a job offer and arrive on the scene.

Academic office space is another story. You may share an office with one or more other faculty or you may have your own four walls. Does your office have a window, proper ventilation, or room for a small conference table? If you are applying for an academic position, I suggest that you ask the chair (or whoever is managing the recruitment) to show you exactly where your office will be.

Once you know about your office, be careful to assure that you will have the equipment you will need, especially what will be required to produce scholarship. Insist on an up-to-date computer, not a "hand-me-down" several years old. A high-speed Internet connection is a must, as is access to clinical records from your academic desk. If you are already engaged in scholarship, ask about the programs you will require: These may include a statistics package, a reference manager such as EndNotes, and a medical spell checker such as Stedman's Plus Medical/Pharmaceutical Spellchecker.[15]

Administrative Support

Access to an administrative assistant (AA) is important as you undertake preparing grants, conducting research, and writing for publication. It is especially helpful if your assigned AA has some skills and experience in scholarly endeavors.

Be prepared to share your AA with others. Typically, a single AA is assigned to work for three or four junior faculty, which creates some competition for time and attention to tasks. If you find that you are sharing an AA with others, I urge you to meet from time to time with your colleagues and work out a plan to share administrative resources and get everyone's work done on the most appropriate schedule.

What do I mean about sharing administrative resources? The following are examples of some agreements that others and I have worked out in the past when we had only one AA to support several faculty members:

- It is not the AA's job to run your personal errands. Do these yourself.
- All typing and similar paperwork should be submitted in folders, and must include a "must-be-completed-by" date. These dates must be realistic and should seldom be "by the end of the day" or *stat*.
- If a job is very urgent, submit it in a red folder. Then red folders get top priority. Red folders should be used very sparingly, and the "red folder prerogative" must not be abused.
- Plan your work well in advance. Do not plan on our AA working overtime in the evenings just because you failed to plan ahead.

Because of computers, faculty today are not as dependent on administrative support as in the past. Nevertheless, computers cannot do your appointment scheduling, photo-copying, mailing, and the many other tasks that you do not need to do personally. So, get the best administrative assistance possible, and be very respectful of this person.

Time for Research and Scholarship

Some new faculty members request "protected research time." In most instances, this is not possible, simply because tight department budgets require that every working hour be productive in some (financial) way. There are instances, however, in which you might be able to negotiate some research time that is not grant funded, at least for a year or two.

It goes like this (one more example of how academic medicine is often an entrepreneurial endeavor). For one reason or another, your and the department chair believe that you have the potential to be a successful grant-writer and researcher. You may then propose the following: You will be allowed a day or two a week to develop your idea and get grant funding. The agreement will have a firm deadline. At the end of the time, you must be on grant funding for your research time or you will return to patient care, and you will be unlikely to succeed with a similar proposal in the future.

Teaching Opportunities

Contact with students is an important benefit of the job. Sadly, many find that teaching time takes us away from patient care and hence reduces take-home income at the end of the month.

One answer may lie in understanding the department's base budget and your own base salary. It is likely that some component of your salary comes from the dean and is intended to support teaching. Do your best to work with your chair to determine what part of your effort allocation is intended for teaching students. Then be sure to sign up for teaching assignments for every hour of this time.

Travel Time and Allowance

Each department seems to handle travel time and funding differently. Some departments and some schools allow 5–10 days each year for professional travel; that is, time to attend medical meetings. The purpose is twofold. First is the necessity of keeping up to date as a clinician. Second is the opportunity to advance professionally by presenting scientific papers or, perhaps, by seeking elected office or serving on national committees.

Funds to travel to meetings generally come from practice income. In some departments, the amounts allowed vary by total clinical income, academic productivity, full-time equivalent time, or the individual's negotiating skills. In our department, we have held that if you are invited to present a research paper, we will find a way to get you to the meeting—if you have proved judicious in how you have used your other travel funds.

PROMOTION AND TENURE

Promotion and tenure (P&T) are the most misunderstood of the academic rewards. In Chapter 2, I described academic faculty ranks and tenure, telling what they mean. Here I will tell how to move up the academic ladder from one rank to another.

To review briefly, the academic ranks are instructor, assistant professor, associate professor, and professor. Tenure, the more-or-less assurance of continued employment and hence the freedom to pursue academic interests without worrying about leadership change or shifting political winds, is a somewhat separate issue.

Being an academic clinician poses special challenges when it comes to promotion and tenure. Academic clinicians focus most of their energy on patient care and teaching—at least they do so early in their careers. I urge that before many years go by, academic clinicians identify a career topic (see Chapter 5) and get started in research and writing. Adding this third skill of the triple-threat academician will make promotion and tenure much more achievable.

The Promotion and Tenure Process

Your plans for promotion (and perhaps tenure) must begin on the day you start your academic career. This means that you should document everything you do in regard to scholarship, teaching, and service, which includes clinical care. You must establish and maintain a curriculum vitae (CV) (see Chapter 4) and you must keep files of every abstract printed, research paper presented, scholarly article published, and any evaluation form, thank-you note, or commendation received. Preserving these items is vital to your promotion, because they will form the basis of your promotion packet—described a little later in this chapter.

What I describe next is necessarily quite general because of the many idiosyncrasies of P&T policies in each medical school.

The Time Line

In most instances, your initial appointment will be at the instructor or assistant professor level—ranks termed "junior faculty." Your goal is to move to "senior faculty" status—associate professor and, eventually, professor.

Each department is likely to have P&T policies that guide the timing and identify the criteria for faculty advancement. Each medical school definitely has such policies. These policies may state, for instance, that advancement from instructor to assistant professor may occur after the individual has been at the instructor rank for at least 2 years and has shown evidence of scholarly productivity and promise.

In many institutions, the chair can appoint an individual at the instructor or assistant professor level, without recourse to the school of medicine's P&T committee. Experienced chairs will seek the approval of the departmental P&T committee prior to any advancement at the junior faculty level and perhaps even before any initial appointments.

The move from assistant to associate professor rank generally becomes reasonable after the faculty member has been an assistant professor for 5–7 years. Many schools require that faculty be actively considered for promotion at the end of 7 years.

Advancement from associate professor to professor is, predictably, the most difficult. Again, it is unlikely to occur until the faculty member has been at the associate professor level for at least 5 years. In some instances, the interval is much longer. In some instances, a faculty member never advances beyond the associate professor level, which then becomes that individual's "terminal rank."

Decisions

The decision to become a candidate for advancement is shared by the departmental P&T committee, the chair, and the faculty member. In the ideal setting, all agree. It is possible for a faculty member to challenge a departmental P&T committee or chair decision to "wait another year," but this is usually a bad idea.

The departmental P&T committee plays a major role in your advancement. The best departmental P&T committees provide faculty members with an annual assessment of their progress toward promotion, identifying areas (typically scholarship) where more effort is needed. Also, when the time comes to be a candidate for promotion, the departmental P&T committee will provide a letter of support and should help you prepare a packet to support your candidacy for promotion.

The school of medicine or the university P&T committee makes the big decision. I don't call it the final decision, because the dean can reverse the decision of an institutional P&T committee and sometimes will actually do so when it is considered in the best interest of the school.

The institutional P&T committee will review the submitted portfolio (the portfolio is described later in this chapter). Someone on the committee will be appointed to review your portfolio in depth and present it to the group, following much the same process as in a grant review (see Chapter 6). In the end, the committee makes a yes-or-no decision, which is submitted to the dean. As an interesting aside: In medical schools, a number of members of your institutional P&T committee will be basic scientists, whose world view and values are much different from those of you—the academic clinician.

Promotion Criteria

As the process begins, your departmental P&T committee will examine your curriculum vitae and compare it to the departmental criteria for advancement. If they give the go-ahead and the chair agrees, then you become a candidate for advancement and the next hurdle is the institutional criteria.

Because of the variety of disciplines of candidates, institutional criteria for promotion to senior faculty ranks are somewhat vague. Here are those for my medical school:[16]

■ Associate Professor: This rank is a senior faculty rank requiring evidence of substantial accomplishment beyond the training and qualifications for appointment to the Assistant Professor rank. Those who aspire to this rank must have a *satisfactory* record of accomplishment in all of the following categories: teaching, scholarship, and service; and a *substantial* record in at least one of these categories.

■ Professor: The rank of Professor is the highest academic rank. It is reserved for appointment or promotion of persons who show clear evidence of a high level of professional accomplishment. Those who aspire to this rank must have a *substantial* record of accomplishment in at least two of the following categories: teaching, scholarship, or service; and an *outstanding* record in the third. Faculty members at or appointed to this rank should have achieved national or international recognition as academicians.

About Tenure

Promotion is about rank, which is—in the end—honorific. That is, there is little or no money attached to the advancement in rank. Tenure is different in that there is the explicit or implicit promise of continued employment, and that may have financial implications for the institution. For this reason, tenure in academic medical centers is granted quite judiciously. Many institutions are currently reexamining their tenure policies and taking steps to reduce the number of tenured faculty.[17]

Here is what my medical school's policy states about tenure for clinicians[16]:

■ Indefinite Tenure—Clinical Science Faculty: The recommendation for award of Indefinite Tenure for clinical faculty requires a documented record of continuous productivity, achieving a level of *outstanding* accomplishment in one of the 3 categories (scholarly activity, teaching and/or service), *substantial* in another and at least *satisfactory* in the third.

In many instances, a faculty member will request both promotion to a senior faculty rank and award of tenure at the same time. The institutional P&T committee may award one—usually the promotion—and not the other.

Most schools have both tenure and nontenure tracks, sometimes called the research and clinical tracks. If you are on a nontenure track, you are not likely to be eligible for tenure in the future, although sometimes it is possible to switch from a nontenure to a tenure track. The ticket to make the switch is scholarly activity—especially grant-funded research and publications in peer-reviewed publications.

Promotion and Tenure: Frequently Asked Questions

Who Is Responsible for Seeing That I Am Promoted to the Appropriate Rank at the Appropriate Time?

The answer: You are! It is true that your mentor, your chair, and the departmental P&T committee are there to help, but the true responsibility is up to you. You must do the work and see that you have documentation. You are the one that must seek some scholarly publications to fill out your CV. You must pay attention to your years in rank and raise the question of your promotion when the time is right.

Can I Be Promoted with Few or No Scholarly Publications on My Curriculum Vitae?

Promotion without some sort of scholarly work is very difficult. In some institutions it is impossible today. In an interesting study of promotion criteria, Gjerde and Colombo asked department chairs and faculty to identify the academic activities most important for promotion.[18] The two groups remarkably agreed on the two top items in their lists:

1. Be primary author of a journal article.
2. Publish articles in refereed journals.

In a study of academic promotion at Johns Hopkins University School of Medicine, Batshaw and colleagues found that, "Those who were promoted had about twice as many articles published in peer-reviewed journals as those who were not promoted."[19]

   Attempting to attain promotion without scholarship is counter to the culture of the institution and is likely to fail. For the academic clinician, scholarship can take the form of "seeking, weighing, formulating, reformulating, and communicating knowledge of clinical practice or teaching."[20]

   My institution, which does not have a "clinical" promotion track, has dealt with the issue by developing an "expanded definition of scholarly activities and service for faculty who engage in clinical activities."[16]

Should I Seek Promotion Early?

In the words of Clint Eastwood as Dirty Harry: "Do you feel lucky?" Maybe you just want to see what happens.

   I strongly discourage this risk-taking. For more than 25 years, I have helped young faculty members decide about becoming promotion candidates, request their support letters, prepare their portfolios, and await the decision of the P&T committee and dean. All this is a process that takes up to a year!

   In the beginning, there is a sense of, "Sure, let's do it. I hope I get promoted, but it will be okay if I am not." After 6 to 8 months of soliciting letters of support from your close friends and colleagues both within your institution and across the country, and then by compiling a packet of up to 200 pages, you have come to take the project very seriously. By now your ego is highly invested. At this point, to be turned down for promotion would be a severe blow to your self-esteem. If unsuccessful, you might conclude, "This school does not respect me or what I do. If they aren't going to promote me and this is what they think of me, I'm going to look around for a job somewhere else."

What About "Up-or-Out" Policies?

In the past, some schools have had an "up-or-out" policy. This generally means that one must be promoted or achieve tenure by 7 years or else be fired. The policy was intended to promote excellence in teaching and other measures of faculty performance and was based on the premise of base salary funding of salaries. The number of years might be different, and there might be various qualifications in different institutions, but you get the gist of the policy.

Not many of these policies exist today, at least in their original form. The rules are changing for several reasons. Grants—euphemistically called "soft money"—cannot be counted on from year to year, and hence institutions would be foolish to "tenure" salaries with soft money. Patient care income can fluctuate considerably from year to year. Some believe that tenure can decrease faculty motivation to teach and conduct research. Thus, as stated by Liu, "Schools have lengthened probationary periods, revised up-or-out provisions, instituted stopping-the-tenure clock policies and less-than-full-time appointments, and permitted faculty to switch between the tenure and non-tenure tracks."[21] One example is a proposed "mommy tenure track" in which primary caregivers of infants are allowed to temporarily postpone their tenure clock.[22]

Getting Academic Clinicians Promoted

A report from Johns Hopkins University School of Medicine states that in their study: "Clinician-educator faculty were less likely to be a higher rank in this institution than were faculty in research paths."[23]

Twenty-five centuries after founding early medical centers and more than 200 years after bring them to America, we are still struggling to bring the awards of academic medicine to those who do the heavy lifting—the physicians who see patients and teach. How can we achieve this goal?

Evidence of change can be found in a paper by Atasoylu and colleagues.[24] In a survey of 114 clinical department chairs compared to an earlier survey of promotion committee chairs, the authors found that "both department chairs and promotion committee chairs value teaching skills and clinical skills as the most important areas of a clinician–educator's performance when evaluating for promotion."

All the above is encouraging for you, the academic clinician. What becomes of practical importance, mindful of lingering biases among the promotion and tenure decision-makers, is how you prepare your promotion portfolio.

Your Academic Promotion Portfolio

According to Simpson and colleagues, "The number of medical schools whose promotion packets include portfolio-like documentation associated with a faculty member's excellence in education has increased by more than 400% in just over ten years."[25] Neglecting to have an academic promotion portfolio is no longer an option for the serious young academic clinician. Table 3.1 presents a list of file folder headings for a model promotion portfolio.

Preparing your academic promotion portfolio has two phases. The first is establishing and maintaining a set of files where you collect every scrap of information that might support your candidacy for promotion. The second phase occurs when you convert these files into a packet to be submitted to the departmental and institutional P&T committees.

In the past, promotion portfolio files have been paper documents. Within a few years, all files and submissions will be electronic. We are now, just as we have been with patient care records, in the awkward transition of switching from paper to computer-based packets. Be wise; plan for the future. In the meantime, you may need to keep duplicate

TABLE 3.1. File folders for your academic promotion portfolio

Personal statement
Curriculum vitae
Position description
Annual performance reviews
Departmental letters
   Department chair
   Departmental P&T committee
Grants written and grants funded
Administrative responsibilities
   Teaching
   Clinical
   Research
Documentation of teaching
   Student teaching
   Resident teaching
   Colleague teaching
Documentation of scholarship (see Chapter 5)
   Discovery
   Clinical activity/application
   Integration
   Teaching
Documentation of continuing education
Special recognition, honors, and awards
Letters of recommendation
   Intrainstitutional
   Extrainstitutional
Best scientific publications

records and perhaps use a scanner to add old documents to your computer's files.

Your academic promotion portfolio should be a living document, with file headings that mirror what will be needed for the final submission packet. Review your portfolio at least annually, and when you receive any sort of documentation of your clinical care, teaching, or scholarship, add it to the files. If in doubt, keep it.

Personal Statement

This will be your rationale for seeking promotion. Organize it in the way that you sense the committee will look at your packet; this is generally in three areas—scholarship, teaching, and service, the latter including clinical care. Then include your list of honors. Most personal statements will be several pages long.

When your packet is considered by the institutional P&T committee, one member of the committee will be tasked to present your qualifications to the group. Bet on the probability that this individual will rely most heavily on what you write in your personal statement. Organize this document carefully and write it very well.

Curriculum Vitae
Keep your latest CV in your promotion portfolio, and update it at least annually. If your school has a required CV format, convert to that model now.

Position Description
This is your official job description, which may also contain your effort allocation—the time, measured in FTE fractions that you theoretically devote to clinical care, teaching, and scholarship.

Annual Performance Reviews
This is the written record of how well you did your job each year. If your department chair is not preparing these for you, request that this be done. You will need these reports at promotion time.

Departmental Letters
When you finally prepare your promotion packet, you will need strong letters of support from your chair and from the departmental P&T committee at that time. I recommend that you supply your chair with an outline of your chief accomplishments organized under the usual headings: scholarship, teaching, and service/clinical. This makes the chair's job much easier and avoids the omission of your best achievements.

Grants Written and Grants Funded
Include all authors/primary investigators, funding agencies, and dollar awards. State clearly who was the lead author or principal investigator.

Administrative Responsibilities
Keep track of all your administrative duties performed over the years.

Documentation of Teaching
Aside from listing courses where you taught, documenting teaching excellence has proved to be difficult. To provide evidence that you have done a good job teaching, save every learner evaluation form and every thank-you note that you receive.

Documentation of Scholarship
Here is where things get interesting for academic clinicians. Medical schools are increasingly recognizing the "scholarship of clinical activity" (sometimes called the "scholarship of application") and "scholarship of teaching." Some items representing clinical activity/application scholarship are listed in Table 3.2. For topics to include under "scholarship of teaching," see Table 3.3.

Documentation of Continuing Education
Your personal continuing medical education (CME) record may or may not be needed for promotion, but you must keep these records somewhere.

TABLE 3.2. Items to consider as scholarship of clinical activity/application

Participation in multicenter collaborative studies
Clinical reports of medical diseases and treatments
Invited clinical lectures
Invited consultations with other institutions
Invited consultations with government agencies
Visiting professorships
Patient education materials
Published clinical observations
Documentation of organizational innovations
Documentation of clinical innovations
Quality assurance documents
Presentations to peers of novel synthesis of knowledge or new clinical techniques
Service as editorial board member or journal reviewer
Participation in national credentialing activities

TABLE 3.3. Items to consider as scholarship of teaching

Educational curricula and courses designed
Introduction of novel techniques for learning
Development of methods to evaluate learning
Course syllabi prepared
Teaching materials
Invited educational lectures
Published pedagogical observations
Computer software for teaching and evaluation
Teaching videos
Educational topic reviews

Special Recognition, Honors and Awards

This includes Alpha Omega Alpha (AOA) membership, teaching awards received from student and residents, awards from your specialty society, and so forth.

Letters of Recommendation

You will not request support letters until you are preparing your packet for submission. At that time, you will need letters from colleagues in your own medical school and those in other institutions. The latter are especially important to establish your regional or national reputation. The rules regarding letters vary; my institution permits candidates for promotion to request a number of support letters and then select the best ones to submit.

Your institution may also require "referee letters," from academicians who do not know you personally. Your chair or mentor should help by supplying a list of names and, probably, by requesting the letters.

Best Scientific Publications

Save copies of these articles when they are published. They may later be sent along with requests for "external referee" letters. A few of the best publications may also be included with your promotion packet, depending on the custom of your school.

TABLE 3.4. Where to learn more about academic medical centers, promotion, and tenure

---

Articles and books

Beasley BW, Wright SM. Looking forward to promotion: characteristics of participants in the Prospective Study of Promotion in Academia. J Gen Intern Med 2003;18:705–710.

Fincher RE, Simpson DE, Mennin SP, et al. Scholarship in teaching: an imperative for the 21st century. Acad Med 2000;75:887–894.

Glick TH. How best to evaluate clinician-educators and teachers for promotion? Acad Med 2002;77:392–397.

Knapper C, Cranton P, eds. Fresh approaches to the evaluation of teaching. New directions for teaching and learning. San Francisco: Jossey-Bass, 2001.

McCabe LRB, McCabe ER. How to succeed in academics. New York: Academic Press, 2000.

Seldin P. The teaching portfolio: a practical guide to improved performance and promotion/tenure decisions, Second ed. Bolton, MA: Anker Publishing, 1997.

Simpson D. The educator's portfolio and CV. Madison: Medical College of Wisconsin, 2002.

Web sites

Association of American Medical Colleges. Medical schools in the U.S. and Canada—alphabetical listing. Available at http://www.aamc.org/members/listings/msalphaae.htm/.

Association of American Medical Colleges. Faculty affairs in academic medicine; selected bibliography. Available at http://www.aamc.org/members/facultyaffairs/bibliography/policyappointmentms.pdf/.

Kuhn G. The educator's portfolio. Available at http://www.saem.org/facdev/FD_manual_2001/educatorkuhn.htm/.

HOW TO LEARN MORE ABOUT ACADEMIC MEDICAL CENTERS

In addition to the reference citations listed at the end of this chapter, you can learn more about AMCs, promotion, and tenure by consulting the sources listed in Table 3.4.

THE UNWRITTEN RULES OF ACADEMIC MEDICAL CENTERS

So far, this chapter has presented beliefs and facts probably well-known to experienced academicians (but not always by junior faculty.) Most of what I presented above can be found in written documents somewhere in the medical center, if you only know where to look. Even the opinions expressed, such as the value system described, can be supported in writing in sometimes-dusty rules and regulations and also in the references cited at the end of the chapter.

But there is more. Academic medicine is "clubby," and there are definitely some unwritten rules of the game. Sometimes these even take the form of "quiet little secrets." In compiling this book, I asked our colleagues, "What are the important unwritten rules in academia?" Here are some of the replies. Note that there are some differing opinions.

- "It is actually dangerous to make an administrative decision around here without checking with everyone, and that means everyone you can think of as a possible stakeholder. Otherwise you are sure to step on someone's toes."
- "I have learned that, if I have an innovative project that I can do on my own without harming anyone, I just go ahead and do it. Rarely does anyone complain. But if I had asked everyone if it was okay, I would never have gotten anything done."
- "Try to have your office and clinical practice 'on-campus.' Being located off campus makes it difficult to attend events and to rub shoulders with department and university leaders."
- "Never attack a fellow faculty member personally. You will probably both be around for a long time, and memory can be long. On the other hand, it is fair game to challenge ideas; that's what academic freedom is about."
- "Pick your collaborators carefully."
- "There is a boundary between teaching faculty and administration. When one assumes an administrative leadership position, they have crossed a line—sometimes referred to by the faculty as going over to the 'dark side.'"
- "Respect the scientists' time. Understand that they are 100% dependent on outside funding and have no other way to support their salaries other than grant and contracts."
- "Make the institution look good."

- "Loyalty to administrative leaders is important and a key to success in climbing the academic ladder."
- "Do the work you are assigned to do, but also figure out a way to get your name on publications."
- "Recognize that one's role in academics is defined by salary and resources, with constant pressure to publish, get funding, and move into leadership."
- "Karma: What you say about someone else *will* get back to you."
- "Be a team player."
- "The faculty do have power in a department, but it is not a good idea to get too far out in front."
- "Learn to put up with unpleasant associates and prima donnas."
- "Make your opportunities; they won't be given to you."
- "Make friends whenever you can, but don't be taken advantage of."
- "Recognize that work hours often extend beyond the 'duty-day,' especially when working on time-sensitive projects with deadlines, like grant proposals."
- "By having two work areas—clinical and academic—it is actually possible to hide from work. I don't recommend it, but it can be done."
- "Get your own money and you can do what you want."
- "The most important unwritten rules are simple—don't give up, don't quit."

WHAT'S NEXT?

Now that you know about the academic medical center's history, organizational structure, and function, Chapter 4 tells how to find the academic job you want.

REFERENCES

1. Phase II Stark Regulations. McDermott Will & Emery. Available at http://www.mwe.com/index.cfm/.
2. Aaron HJ. Policy Brief #59: The plight of academic medical centers. Washington, DC: The Brookings Institution, 2000.

3. Sebastian A. The dictionary of the history of medicine. New York: Pantheon, 1999, p. 7.

4. Asimov I. Beginnings—the history of mankind, life, the earth, the universe. New York: Berkley, 1987, p. 55.

5. Bordley J, Harvey AM. Two centuries of American medicine. Philadelphia: Saunders, 1976, pp. 10–11.

6. Flexner A. Medical education in the United States and Canada. New York: Carnegie Foundation for the Advancement of Teaching, 1910.

7. Janeway CA. The decline of primary medical care: an unforeseen consequence of the Flexner Report. The Pharos 1974; July: 74–78.

8. Beck AH. The Flexner Report and the standardization of American medical education. JAMA 2004;291:2139–2140.

9. Taylor RB. Family medicine: now and future practice. In: Family medicine: principles and practice, 6th ed. Taylor RB, ed. New York: Springer-Verlag, 2003, pp. 3–9.

10. Rankings of Top Medical Schools, Research and Primary Care. U.S. News and World Report. Available at http://www.usnews.com/usnews/edu/grad/rankings/med/medindex_brief.php.

11. Begus GR, Randall CS, Winniford MD, Mueller CW, Johnson SR. Job satisfaction and workplace characteristics of primary and specialty care physicians at a bimodal medical school. Acad Med 2001;76:1148–1152.

12. Ruedy J, MacDonald NE, MacDougall B. Ten-year experience with mission-based budgeting in the faculty of medicine of Dalhousie University. Acad Med 2003;78:1121–1129.

13. Applegate WB, Williams ME. Career development in academic medicine. Am J Med 1990;88:263–267.

14. Hafler JP, Lovejoy FH, Jr. Scholarly activities recorded in the portfolios of teacher-clinician faculty. Acad Med 2000;75: 649–652.

15. Taylor RB. The clinician's guide to medical writing. New York: Springer-Verlag, 2005.

16. Guidelines for promotion and tenure for primary faculty of the school of medicine. Portland, OR: Oregon Health & Science University, November 2, 2000.

17. Halpern EC. Is tenure irrelevant for academic clinicians? South Med J 1995;88:1099–1106.

18. Gjerde CL, Colombo DE. Promotion criteria: perceptions of faculty members and departmental chairmen. J Med Educ 1982;57:157–162.

19. Batshaw ML, Plotnick LP, Petty BG, Wolff PK, Mellits ED. Academic promotion at a medical school. Experience at

Johns Hopkins University School of Medicine. N Engl J Med 1988;318:741–747.

20. Lubitz RM. Guidelines for promotion of clinician-educators. J Gen Intern Med 1997;12:S71–S77.

21. Liu M, Mallon WT. Tenure in transition: trends in basic science faculty appointments policies at U.S. medical schools. Acad Med 2004;79:205–213.

22. Draznin J. The "mommy tenure track." Acad Med 2004; 79:289–290.

23. Thomas PA, Diener-West M, Canto MI, Martin DR, Post WS, Streiff MB. Results of an academic promotion and career path survey of faculty at the Johns Hopkins University School of Medicine. Acad Med 2004;79:258–264.

24. Atasoylu AA, Wright SM, Beasley BW, et al. Promotion criteria for clinician-educators. J Gen Intern Med 2003;18:711–716.

25. Simpson D, Hafler J, Brown D, Wilkerson L. Documentation systems for educators seeking academic promotion in U.S. medical schools. Acad Med 2004;79:783–790.

4
Finding the Academic Job You Want

If, after learning about academic careers and academic medical centers (AMCs), you decide that becoming an academic clinician is right for you, your next step is a careful search for the position you want and that is right for you. I hope that these two positions are the same, but such is not always the case.

You need to identify the best fit for your skills and temperament and then take the big step into the academic job market. To do this, you will need to have a well-prepared curriculum vitae (CV); you will need to understand the academic recruitment "dance" and how to evaluate an academic job offer; and you will need to know what works and what doesn't when it comes to negotiating your academic employment contract.

Of course, if you are already in an academic faculty position, this chapter will affirm what you did right, reveal what you could have done better, and help you plan for your next job search.

THE RIGHT POSITION FOR YOU

What Is the Right Academic Job for Me?

The right position for you will be a good fit of your abilities with the needs and aspirations of the medical school and the department you might join. A key consideration is the medical school's commitment to your discipline. As I discussed in Chapter 3, medical schools may be considered focused on research productivity or primary care, and a few are considered hybrid schools. Where does your potential employer fit in the scheme? If not clear to you, I would ask during interviews, and I would also check the annual ranking of *U.S. News and World Report*, available at

http://www.usnews.com/usnews/edu/grad/rankings/med/
medindex_brief.php/.

You also need to think about why the medical school is recruiting you. As stated by Applegate and Williams: "If the goals of the institutional leadership appear based on monetary concerns (need to increase clinical revenues by seeing more patients) or fashionable motives (others are developing similar programs and we don't want to be left behind), academic values related to scholarship and teaching may well be compromised over time."[1]

As a junior faculty member, you will have little direct contact with the dean, and your sense of the school's direction and orientation will remain "institutional." Within your own department, however, the issues become more personal.

Medical school departments are highly driven by the values and goals of the department chair. Be sure you meet with this individual, and try to assess if he or she is someone you trust and whose vision matches yours. This is vital because, as stated by one of the book's contributors, "The Department chair has total power over your life." Although the contributor's comment may be a bit hyperbolic, you should look for a department chair who values diverse opinions, open dialogue, and individual growth of faculty. During interviews, be sure to ask junior faculty about these topics.

Another desirable trait in a chair is the willingness to have faculty change roles. This promotes development of new academic skills and can prepare you for advancement. It also avoids departmental ossification, with little or no chance for young faculty to advance.

How Do I Find Out What Jobs Are Available?

Many of the most desirable academic positions are advertised only once, and the notice might be in a journal that you do not read. If the job is really an outstanding opportunity, the department chair may already have a file of potential candidates, including a few "inside" candidates knocking on the door. This means that you must use all available means to find not only the hard-to-fill jobs but also the most promising positions.

What the Contributors Report
The following are what the book's contributors report when asked, "How did you find your first academic position?"

- "I had kept in touch with my best friend from residency. He seemed really happy working in an academic department, and I told him to let me know if anything came available."
- "I answered an ad in JAMA. A lot of other people did also, and I think I was lucky to get the job."
- "My first job was created for me with 'soft money.' Otherwise I would have been in private practice."
- "I was recruited out of residency."
- "I took a research fellowship after residency. My fellowship training made me very attractive to potential employers. I would not have the job I have now if I had not done a research fellowship."
- "I sent out a letter and résumé to academic departments in the region of the country I was interested in."
- "I found out about the position through word of mouth and then applied. I had prepared myself by doing a number of faculty development activities."
- "I actually began preparing myself for it before I even started medical school. As a pre-med student, I began a dialogue with members of the department I was interested in (and where I was ultimately hired). Advice I received from the chair of the department, among others, helped me chart a course through medical school and residency."

Sources of Information About Academic Positions
If you are looking for an academic position, you need to use every resource available so that you can make the best choice of which opportunities to investigate. Your mentor or a senior faculty member is a great place to start. This person knows the recruitment process and probably has some useful contacts that may yield a list of promising openings. I recommend that you talk with your mentor first.

Check with your national specialty society. Many have divisions that deal with academics, and these divisions may maintain a file of available positions. Call the specialty society by telephone, and explain what you are seeking.

Contact your contemporaries whose academic careers have taken them to other institutions. This is an good opportunity to renew old acquaintances.

Finally, there is the traditional way to search for a job—classified advertisements. Almost all specialty journals have listings of open positions, which will include some academic opportunities. Also look in the major broad-based medical journals: the *Journal of the American Medical Association* (JAMA) and in the *New England Journal of Medicine* (NEJM). You might review a copy of *Academic Medicine* and look at the positions available in their section "Index of Positions Listed," although many of these notices are for high-level appointments, such as Associate Dean or Chief of a Clinical Department.

I like to do things online; I find the process quick and inexpensive. If you are seeking an academic job, I suggest that you try these Web sites:

- JAMA Career Opportunities Online. Go to http://dbapps.ama-assn.org. Then click on "Classified Ads," and then on "Academic/Faculty."
- The New England Journal Career Center. This is available at http://www.nejmjobs.org
- Academic Physician and Scientist. Begin at http://www.acphysci.com/aps/app. Then click on "Clinical Science," followed by your specialty.
- The Riley Guide: Job Listings in Healthcare and Medical Fields. Go to http://www.rileyguide.com. Then look for "Medical Schools."
- Academic Careers Online. This has listings for a variety of research, scientific, and academic vacancies. Check out http://www.academiccareers.com/.
- MedCentener Today. Go to http://www.medcentertoday.com. Then look for the section: "MedCenter Jobs Online."

How Do I Let It Be Known That I Am Looking for an Academic Position?

Networking

You start a job search by networking. Tell all your friends and professional contacts that you are available for the right academic position. You will, of course, focus your effort on colleagues already in academia and especially in those schools and departments that your research has identified as potential good fits for you.

Letters of Inquiry

Next, consider sending letters of inquiry to the chairs of selected departments. I recommend a one-page letter indicating your interest in an academic position and why you plan this career move. Be sure to tell any special interests or skills you have—such as sports medicine experience, a Certificate of Added Qualifications in Geriatrics, foreign language skills, a specific surgical ability, and so forth. Specify whether or not this inquiry is confidential (see below). Then add a current copy of your curriculum vitae and send it out.

I spent 14 years as chairman of an academic clinical department, and during this time, I kept an active file of unsolicited letters of interest in jobs that might become available in the department. When a position became open, I checked the file for possible candidates.

Association of American Medical Colleges (AAMC) Job Board

The AAMC Job Board is an online forum for medical schools and prospective faculty candidates. Job seekers can find information about available positions and can post their CVs for review by prospective employers. The Web site is http://www.aamc.org/jobboard/start.htm/.

Personal Advertisement

Should you run your own advertisement in a medical journal? "Skilled clinician seeks academic position involving teaching and scholarship." In the usual course of academic recruitment, this is seldom done. That does not make a personal classified advertisement a bad idea; it only means that most job applicants don't think of it. If you decide to do so, I suggest you start with the journals and Web sites listed above.

CONFIDENTIALITY IN THE JOB SEARCH

In academic medicine, a setting in which successful departments sometimes attempt to lure valued faculty away from departments at other institutions, the issue of confidentiality is critical. If you state early on that your inquiry is confidential, the chair will respect this. A common way to avoid tying the hands of the chair you hope will hire you is to have a short list of individuals that know about your search and that will serve as confidential references.

On the other hand, if you specify that the search is not confidential and if the chair likes your inquiry letter and CV, he or she may call your residency director or someone else who might reasonably have an opinion to ask about you. Remember that medicine, and especially academic medicine, is a surprisingly small family.

As chairman, and later as professor emeritus acting for the chairman, I have made telephone calls about persons who sent a job application or an unsolicited inquiry letter, often contacting my acquaintances whom I suspected might know the applicant. If I discovered red flags during my phone conversations, the recruitment was unlikely to continue. And in most instances, the applicant never knew that inquiries were made.

HOW TO PREPARE A CURRICULUM VITAE

In academics and also in business, there is a truism: Your record gets you the interview; your interview gets you the job. Hence your curriculum vitae (I have also seen the document called a curriculum vita and will leave this debate to Latin scholars) is a crucial document, as this presents the details of your "life record."

The CV is a comprehensive, biographical listing of your professional activities, including your education and training, academic appointments, publications, and more; the older you are, the longer your CV is likely to become. A CV is similar to a résumé but differs in several key ways: First of all, a CV is intended to be comprehensive and detailed. In constructing a CV, the general rule is, "If you wonder if it should be included, put it in." In contrast, a résumé is generally brief and may be as short as two pages.

Second, the CV is a formal list of past activities and achievements, whereas a résumé may tell your objective (e.g., to secure a position that utilizes your special talents, which you will go on to describe). Also, a résumé may tell specific details about the jobs you have held, such as the number of persons you supervised or the size of the budget you managed. All academicians need an up-to-date CV. For the academician, a separate résumé is generally unnecessary.

Format and Content of Your Curriculum Vitae

There is no set format to a curriculum vitae.[2] With that said, however, some institutions have prescribed formats. For example, the University of Toronto has a good one that is available online.[3] My medical school insists that all candidates for promotion submit their CVs in a very specific outline. Table 4.1 presents a useful format for a CV.

Principles of Writing Your Curriculum Vitae

Writing a CV is a learned skill. The following are some principles that can make the task a little easier and help assure a better document.

Consistency

It is easy to become inconsistent in various aspects of your CV, for the simple reason that things are added incrementally. With each new invited lecture, paper, or grant award, you make an entry. Be sure that all entries are uniform as to headings, font, punctuation, and citation style.

TABLE 4.1. A basic curriculum vitae topic outline

Professional and personal information: For security reasons, do not list your social security number.

Education: Begin with college and tell all education and training, including academic degrees awarded.

Professional experience: Where have you worked? Again, include dates.

Professional certification: Are you board-certified in your specialty?

Licensure: List all states in which you hold a current medical license.

Professional society memberships: Tell national and state organizations and any leadership roles you have held. Include dates.

Honors and awards: Include Phi Beta Kappa or Alpha Omega Alpha, teaching awards, and any other formal recognition.

Grants and contracts: Tell the grant titles, funding agencies and dollar amounts of awards.

Publications: List all, categorized by peer-reviewed journals, non–peer-reviewed journals, books, book chapters, and other publications. Use the citation format recommended by the International Committee of Medical Journal Editors (ICMJE)[4]

Teaching: Describe courses you have taught and include the institution and when you taught them.

Service: Tell about service to your community, which might include volunteer work or participation in service organizations.

Invited presentations: Here is where you list lectures you were asked to present at state, regional, or national meetings or at other medical centers.

Chronological Order

In the CV, you will be making lists of items in various categories: (see Table 4.1). Be sure that you choose one chronological style and stick to it. I prefer to present my papers, lectures, and so forth in reverse order—with the latest publication at the top of the list. Unless your university has a required chronological style, it probably doesn't matter as long as you are consistent throughout the document.

Abbreviations

Abbreviations are conveniences that often confuse and mislead. I recommend using no abbreviations on your CV. If you must use an abbreviation, you should explain its use the first time it appears on the document. But remember that someone looking at your CV may be skipping back and forth and not reading it like a book chapter. Thus the person evaluating you for a job or for promotion may miss the explanation that OSU means Ohio State University and not Oklahoma State University, that HRSA means Health Resources and Services Administration, or that your invited lecture on TD was on tardive dyskinesia and not on travelers' diarrhea.

White Space

Use generous spacing on your CV. There is no reason to crowd the page. Use 12-point font, and arrange items in a visually pleasing manner. Review the CVs of some successful faculty to see how they have arranged items.

Accuracy

Be sure your CV is absolutely accurate and not misleading in any way. Include nothing that could be misread in a way that might undermine your credibility.

Red Flags

Table 4.2 tells items on a CV that may concern a potential employer or raise questions when you are considered for promotion.

CV Maintenance

Your CV is a living document. Be sure to keep it up to date. I do so by maintaining a "CV Update" file. When I publish a paper or present a lecture, I drop a copy of the paper or the meeting program in the file. Every 4–6 months, I take out the CV and add the items in the folder.

TABLE 4.2. Red flags on a curriculum vitae

Carelessness: Misspellings, grammatical errors, handwritten corrections, general sloppiness.

Out of date: Failure to reflect recent changes in status or accomplishments.

Unexplained time periods: Were you in jail or a drug rehabilitation center during the undocumented time?

Exaggerations: If you were the fifth co-investigator on a large grant, don't write the CV entry to look as though you were the leader of the project.

Cuteness: Do not tell about your skills in winemaking or your love of hip-hop music; you are preparing a professional document.

Consider making an abbreviated CV. As your CV gets longer and longer, create a one-page CV. Mine contains personal information, education and training, honors and awards, professional memberships, and a total number of my research papers, book chapters, and books published.

Be sure that your CV and your abbreviated CV are available on your computer. When you need to send a CV, it is often most convenient to do so as an e-mail attachment.

RECRUITMENT

You have done your research about a specific academic position, polished your CV, and contacted the department chair. The position is still open and the department is interested in you as a candidate. The recruitment dance begins.

Actually, recruitment is much like courtship. It is enjoyable, everyone is exhibiting best behavior, but the end may not be a long-term relationship.

What Academic Departments Are Looking for in an Applicant

In addition to filling identified clinical needs, such as someone who can perform a key surgical procedure or a doctor with a special certificate of added qualifications, academic departments are typically looking for candidates who possess certain general desirable characteristics. Some of these are listed in Table 4.3.

TABLE 4.3. Attributes desired by academic department chairs

Professional	Personal
Excellent clinical skills	Self-confidence
Ability to fit in with the group	High energy level
Integrity	Motivation
Willingness to work hard	Emotional stability
Reliability	Ability to communicate effectively
Scholarly approach to medicine	Ability to listen attentively

The Interview Visit

Your record got you the interview; now is your time to get the job. You will want to prepare carefully for the interview, stay alert and focused, mind your manners, and finish strong.

Preparing for the Interview

Try to get a copy of your interview schedule ahead of time, and then do some research on everyone you will meet. Look on the medical school Web site, check their names on Google, and look up their papers on the Web at http:www.PubMed.com.

Be sure to find out exactly how to pronounce the names of your interviewers. Smith and Brown are easy. Many names are not. Also be sure to learn the names of the staff persons who will assist with your visit; they can be surprisingly important in influencing department decisions.

Consider coming prepared with written questions, and don't hesitate to refer to your prepared question list during the interview. I view this as a matter of personal style.

Pack an extra copy of your CV and your list of references. If you have written a paper that you are especially proud of, put a copy in your briefcase. Also, bring a blank pad to take notes.

Be prepared to leave with the chair a list of persons who have agreed to serve as references for you. Bring a list to the interview, even if you submitted it earlier with your application packet. I prefer to keep the list separate from my CV. Everyone on your list is likely to be contacted, perhaps when a decision is being made about inviting you to interview but certainly before offering you a position.

Finally, remind yourself that the interview starts the moment you arrive and doesn't end until you are home again. In between, everyone you meet is evaluating your behavior at every minute.

Interview Skills

Begin the interview with a firm, business-like handshake. This is important; a wimpy handshake makes a poor first impression. While shaking hands, look the interviewer in the eye, repeat his or her name, and state that you are glad to meet this person.

Determine where you should sit. I once entered an interviewer's office, shook hands with him and sat in the nearest chair. It wasn't long before I realized that I had sat in the interviewer's desk chair. We had an awkward moment, and then we both moved to sit in the correct seats.

Let the interviewer take the initial lead. Anticipate some questions about your trip or another nonthreatening subject. From there, he or she will go to progressively more focused questions. I will not attempt to anticipate all the questions you may be asked, but I suggest that you practice with someone experienced in interviewing job applicants. The usual questions will be much like those you encountered when interviewing for medical school and residency: What are your strengths and weaknesses? What are you looking for in a job? What abilities will you bring to this job?

Prepare for the "negative" questions that you might be asked. For example:

- Tell me an example of something you have attempted and failed.
- What has been the biggest disappointment in your professional life?
- What sort of professional tasks do you not like to do?
- When is it acceptable to break the rules? When did you last do so?
- When have you benefitted from constructive criticism?

What about the illegal questions? These include queries about marital status, childcare, race or nationality, religion, physical illness or disability, or even birth control. If you suspect that such a question might arise, decide in advance how you will handle the situation. The answer is not easy. You may just answer the question, assuming that the interviewer is not up to date on illegal questions. You and the interviewer move on to another topic, and you are still in the running for the job.

Another approach to the illegal question is to ask your interviewer to explain what your religion, childbearing plans, or personal illness might have to do with the job. Do this in a polite, light-hearted manner, and you may still get the job. If you become outraged and express your anger about the question, you and your interviewer may both decide that this is not the job for you.

While discussing interview behavior, let me list some things not to do:

■ Do not drink more than one cup of coffee during an interview day. It can make you jittery, cause you to talk too much, and send you to the toilet too often.

■ Do not drink alcohol at any time during your interview visit. You will probably be taken to lunch or dinner. Leave the cocktail drinking to others. Keep your head clear.

■ Don't order foods that are difficult to eat. Crab legs and lobster come to mind. Stick with foods that are easy to cut and chew. Do not overeat, especially at lunch. You probably have a busy, intense afternoon ahead and don't want to become drowsy.

■ Do not interrupt. Your interviewer may be long-winded. That is all right, because it takes some pressure off you. Whatever happens, let the interviewer finish speaking before you reply.

■ Don't speak badly about your current colleagues or about other institutions at which you have interviewed or worked. Just as patients who disparage their former doctors make me anxious, experienced academicians know full well that anyone who criticizes others may soon be speaking badly about them.

■ Do not be rude to staff.

■ Don't even think about smoking.

After the Interview

After your academic job interview, do what your mother taught you. Send a personal thank-you note to everyone who interviewed you. Try to make each note personal; if possible, refer to something you discussed during your interview time or at dinner. Also send a thank-you note to your chief contact on the administrative staff whom, I am sure, worked very hard arranging your visit.

Then wait, at least for a reasonable time, which may be 2 or 3 weeks. The department may be interviewing others before making a decision. At this time the ball is on their side of the net. If you have heard nothing by the end of 3 weeks, you might reasonably call to request an update on progress with the search.

THE ACADEMIC JOB OFFER AND CONTRACT

If recruitment is a type of courtship, then a job offer is like a marriage proposal—a bid to link destinies in a long-term relationship. If things have gone well between you and the department, here will be an offer, probably some negotiation, and then a signed agreement.

The Offer and the Contract

The initial job offer is most likely to be verbal, either in a face-to-face meeting or on the telephone. This allows each party to test the reactions of the other and to get a sense of how much negotiation will be needed to get to "yes."

If you and the person making the offer reach general agreement on role, duties, and salary, then the next step will be an offer letter. This letter is what spells out the conditions of your employment. You may receive a preprinted appointment acknowledgment from the university's central administration, but the offer letter is what binds you and the academic department. Almost certainly the letter you receive has been reviewed and approved by the dean's office, and it carries the weight of a formal contract. Table 4.4 tells the basic components of an offer letter.

Negotiation

Some items in the offer letter are negotiable; almost everything in the offer letter is open to discussion. If an item, such as starting faculty rank, was previously discussed verbally and if you and the chair (or designee) reached agreement, then renegotiating at a later time is really not playing fairly.

TABLE 4.4. Basic components of an offer letter for an academic position

Your name and address. Be sure that this letter was intended for you and not someone else. Stranger things have happened.

Identification of the position. Often this will relate to a separate document, the position description (see Chapter 2).

Full-time equivalent (FTE). If anything less than 1.0 FTE, be sure you understand the reasons and the implications.

Starting faculty rank. This will be instructor, assistant professor, (possibly) associate professor, or (highly unlikely) professor. There may also be a modifier, such as "clinical" or "adjunct" (see Chapter 2).

Starting salary. What will you be paid? Generally this is stated as a yearly salary.

Start date. When are you expected to report for work?

Moving expenses. You may be offered up to 10% of the starting base salary.

Special expectations or requirements. For example, you may be formally encouraged to take an active role in your local and state specialty organization.

Special restrictions. This may include prohibitions against practicing outside the medical center ("moonlighting") or locating a practice within a certain radius of the medical center if you cease employment (restrictive covenant).

Basic Benefits. Some items won't be in the offer letter, but you need to know about them. Some important ones are listed in Table 4.5.

But if an issue, such as a restrictive covenant, was not previously discussed, you may question the issue after the offer letter arrives. Remember that what you hold in your hand is a letter prepared by word processing on a computer; it is not technically difficult to modify the document.

In my opinion, your most important issue is your time allocation. If an academic position is 90–100% patient care, is it much different than private practice? Aim for at least 0.1 to 0.2 full-time equivalent (FTE) for teaching or scholarship. More is better if you can get it.

Your power in negotiation comes, of course, from how badly the department wants to hire you. If you are one of four very similar candidates for the job and have no special abilities that the department needs, your negotiating potential is limited. On the other hand, if you have a special skill or if you come bringing grant support, then you are in a stronger bargaining position. This brings me to a useful saying when applying for a job: "You make your deals on the doorstep." This means that your most favorable negotiating time is before your sign the offer letter. Once you have agreed to the offer in writing, the time for negotiation has passed.

Here are comments on a few of the items in Table 4.5, which lists what you should learn before accepting a job

TABLE 4.5. What you need to know about before accepting an academic job offer

---

Roles and duties of the position, including your time and effort allocation to:
    Clinical care
    Teaching
    Research
    Administration
The culture and esprit de corps of the academic department
Access to administrative assistance and computer support
Office location: Where will you have a desk?

Health benefits:
    Health insurance, including hospitalization
    Dental insurance
    Prescription drug insurance

Other benefits:
    Vacation
    Educational leave and travel funds available
    Sick-leave policy
    Family-medical leave policy
    Association dues
    Life insurance
    Disability insurance
Retirement plan, such as a 401k, 403b, 457, or other deferred compensation plan

Professional liability insurance:
    Extent of coverage
    Tail coverage
Promotion and tenure
    Will I eventually be eligible for tenure?
    Is there an "up-or-out" policy? (see Chapter 3)
Miscellaneous
    Parking
    Family education benefits
    Outside income restrictions

---

offer. It is very important that you get a true reading on the culture and esprit de corps in the department. Don't be fooled by everyone's "interview behavior" and arrive to find a conflicted group with warring factions.

Be sure to ask the questions: "May I see where my office will be?" And, "Who will provide my administrative support, and how much of this person's time will be available for my work?" You might find that you will be in a shared office. If so, be sure to meet your future office-mate to be sure this is someone with whom you will want to spend a lot of hours working in shared space.

Health benefits are generally not negotiable, but you should find out what options are available.

Ask about vacation, educational leave, and any travel funds available. Also, does the institution or faculty practice plan pay for medical association dues, life insurance or disability insurance, and reference books or journal subscriptions?

Retirement plans may not seem very important when you are young but become of keen interest as you age. At the end of your career, you are likely to find that your greatest financial asset is the money in your retirement plans. Find out what is available from the institution and perhaps from the faculty practice plan. Also, start now to learn about the following plans that might be offered to you[5,6]:

- 401k plan: This is a plan established by an employer to which eligible employees may make salary-deferral (and thus, there is current salary reduction) contributions. In some plans, the employer matches part or all of the employee's contribution. As with the 403b and 457 plans, 401k earnings grow on a tax-deferred basis.
- 403b plan: Certain employees of public schools and other tax-exempt organizations are eligible to participate in 403b plans. Some think of the 403b plan as a 401k plan for employees of public institutions.
- 457 plan: This is a tax-deferred, salary reduction plan for qualified employees of government and non-church-controlled tax-exempt organizations.

Be sure to inquire about professional liability insurance. In most academic jobs, the year-by-year cost is borne by the faculty practice plan or the institution. The big surprise can come when you leave the position and find that you must pay thousands of dollars to buy "tail coverage." Tail coverage is the cost of covering suits that arise after you leave your current job. Be sure to look into this when negotiating for an academic position so that you will not face an unexpected expense when you leave.

One negotiable item may be professional liability tail coverage when you leave a current position and enter academics. In some instances, the department hiring you will pay your tail coverage from a previous practice. Look at it as a signing bonus, even if the money is going to an insurance company and not to you directly.

A faculty member once quipped that a university is a loose federation of departments united by a common parking problem. Where you will park won't be a deal-breaker as far as the job negotiation is concerned, but an enlightened candidate might tactfully inquire.

A few university systems offer discounted tuition to their undergraduate schools for family members. This can be a major benefit to you and your family, especially if you have children who will enter college soon.

If you have any thoughts of moonlighting or working outside the university hospital, inquire about any restrictions. Also, clarify when the university's professional liability plan will cover you and when it won't.

Part-time Work and Job Sharing

What about negotiating for a part-time position? More and more physicians are considering this option, not only as they wind down their careers but also during the child-rearing years and perhaps during midlife. Women physicians pioneered part-time work, but a recent article points out that, "The trend toward fewer hours is gaining momentum as men join in."[7] According to Croasdale, the American Medical Association's Women Physician Congress is accumulating information and resources on the topic. In academic medicine, there seems to be some early efforts to develop part-time faculty tracks. One such effort is at the University of Miami School of Medicine.[7]

If you are considering applying for an advertised full-time position with a proposal to work part-time, I urge you to consider carefully. If you are a highly desirable candidate, especially a proven grant-getter, your suggestion may be seriously considered. On the other hand, if you are applying for a typical clinician-teacher position, with duties that are primarily patient care, an offer to work only part-time may be seen as not making a commitment to your patients and your department. Your colleagues involved in patient care may see your proposal as being a burden to the practice group, especially in regard to after-hours coverage.

If you intend to offer your part-time services in response to an advertised full-time position, be ready to make the case for why the department should make an ongoing investment in you. One small bargaining chip is that if working less than 0.5 FTE, you will probably save your department money: The savings occurs because, when you are only working part-time, the department will probably not be paying for certain fringe benefits for you. Also, "part-time" workers often put in many extra, unpaid hours. In the end, your proposal to join an academic clinical department working part-time will be successful only if they can see why the arrangement is to the department's long-term advantage. It is your responsibility to help them understand why this is so.

Job-sharing is a variant of part-time work in which two persons collaborate to "share" one position. Your institutional policy is likely to consider both as working 0.5 FTE and thus both eligible for full fringe benefits; this is a financial disadvantage to the department and makes job-sharing unattractive to academic employers.

EARLY CAREER ERRORS

In the Preface of this book, I alluded to getting experience by making mistakes. The following are five early career errors made by young academic clinicians.

■ **Taking the wrong job at the wrong department in the wrong institution.** Be sure that you intuitively like the chair or division chief and the individuals who will be your professional colleagues. Be sure that the department's mission is consonant with yours, whether the greatest value is placed on excellence in patient care, teaching, or scholarship. And don't misunderstand the institutional goals and culture; be sure that you can support what seems to be the chief mission—obtaining more and more research grant funding, caring for the underserved, catering to the wealthy elite who may become future donors, teaching students who will be outstanding future physicians, or some other institutional objective.

■ **Taking a job without full support of your spouse and family.** I have been on the faculty of the Oregon Health & Science University for 21 years. I have seen far too many faculty recruited, many at considerable cost, just to see them leave after 6–12 months. Why? Often I discover that the spouse never wanted to move to the new location. In looking back, I sometimes find that there was little involvement of the spouse and family in the recruitment process. In short, the spouse and family did not have a clear picture of the job, the city, the climate, and the culture of Oregon. To avoid the problem of spouse dissatisfaction and losing a valued recruit, I urge that the spouse come along on all recruitment interview trips. If he or she refuses to come or there are indications of reluctance, considerable energy and expense can be avoided.

■ **Taking on too much too soon.** In the beginning, the new faculty member seems to have a lot of free time. There is the tendency, then, for the existing faculty members to recruit the new arrival to this committee and that task force. He or she is invited to take on far too much and happily accepts all the invitations. The opportunities all sound interesting and, as a newcomer, you don't want to offend. Before long, the new faculty member is as overwhelmed as everyone else in the department. A good defensive ploy is to defer accepting any invitations until you have spoken with your mentor or your chair. This gives you time to consider the time commitment and someone else to cite if you decide to say, "No."

■ **Fighting the bureaucracy of the institution.** The institution has more rules and forms than you can imagine. You will need to document "effort" in numerical terms. There is required training in everything from HIPAA (the Health Insurance Portability and Accountability Act of 1996) to how to use the new transcription system. Everything is evaluated. Stalling and stonewalling will do you no good at all. Bureaucracy is part of academic medicine. Learn to love it, or be prepared to suffer what happens to the noncompliant individual in an institutional setting.

■ **Believing that the system will reward you differently than it has dealt with everyone else in the past.** In Chapter 3, I discussed the various rewards of academia—salary, promotion and tenure, teaching opportunities, access to resources, and more. Be sure you clearly understand how these rewards are distributed in your institution and what you will need to do to get your fair share. Ask about how the pie is cut, find out who gets the large pieces and why, and do not expect the system to change for you.

SIGNING THE AGREEMENT AND STARTING YOUR JOB

After learning about AMCs in general and a few in particular, and after applying and interviewing for your dream job, you receive an offer. The terms are right—perhaps following a little negotiation. You sign the agreement and begin your new job. From this point on, you will be expected to acquire some basic academic skills. These include adapting your clinical care to the academic medical center model, learning to be an effective educator, and setting the stage for your personal scholarly activity. As you continue in your career, you will need to learn more advanced academic skills: getting grants, doing research, and writing for publication. Chapter 5 presents an overview of some basic academic skills. In Chapter 6, I will discuss selected important points about the advanced academic skills.

REFERENCES

1. Applegate WB, Williams ME. Career development in academic medicine. Am J Med 1990;88:263–267.
2. Hansen RS. Preparing a curriculum vitae. Available at http://www.quintcareers.com/curriculum_vitae.html.
3. Faculty of Medicine/University of Toronto. CV format. Available at http://www.medicine.facmed.ca/userfiles/HTML/nts_1_725_1.html.
4. International Committee of Medical Journal Editors. Uniform requirements for manuscripts submitted to biomedical journals. Available at http://www.icmje.org/.
5. Retirement plans are explained at http://www.investopedia.com/terms.
6. McKinney HW. Your guide to retirement planning. Available at http://www.retireplan.about.com.
7. Croasdale M. Women physicians find ways to make "part-time" work. Available at http://www.ama-assn.org/amednews/2004/11/15/prl21115.htm/.

5

Basic Academic Skills: Clinical Practice, Teaching, and Scholarship

On any given day, I can watch the news on CNN from morning until bedtime. Or I can watch the news highlights on the "News at Nine" in the evening. Chapters 5 and 6 are like the news highlights. These two chapters on basic and advanced academic skills describe what I think you really need to know albeit admitting that coverage is far short of comprehensive. There are scores of books on teaching, scholarship, grant writing, and the other topics presented, and some of the best sources are listed in tables found in the chapters of this book. I urge you to continue your study of medical academia by reading some of these books, articles, and Web sites.

In the meantime, here are some highlights—an overview—of basic academic skills.

CLINICAL SKILLS

It may seem ironic that I begin my discussion of basic academic skills with a section on clinical skills. After all, aren't your clinical skills exactly what make you an attractive candidate for an academic faculty position?

Of course, your abilities as a clinician were (or will be) key factors in your being hired. However, the quiet little secret is that, as soon as you enter academic medicine, your treasured clinical skills may begin to atrophy. How could this happen? Consider the following: In training you attended educational conferences and treated patients every day. In private practice, except for the occasional hospital committee meeting, you spent almost all your professional time caring for patients and augmenting your clinical expertise.

Academic practice is very different. As an academic clinician, you will have many conflicting duties that include lecturing, leading small-group discussions, attending meetings, writing grants, doing research, and writing papers. All these activities, critical as they are to your academic career, take you away from patient care. Some senior faculty see patients only about 20% of their time, and this is not enough direct patient contact to keep up to date on emerging diagnostic methods, new drugs and doses, and recently developed procedures. Academic clinicians will spend most of their time in clinical care where they often work with residents; their direct patient care time is still a good deal less than it would be in private practice. In short, when you enter academics, you may see your clinical abilities gradually dwindle.

In some specialties, there is an even more pernicious force that can wither clinical skills—supervision of residents performing surgical procedures. Consider that you enter academic medicine able to perform a very capable bowel resection, knee replacement, or cardiac catheterization. In a teaching setting, however, the educational imperative often prompts you to cede the hands-on activity to senior residents and fellows. After a few years, the procedure-based clinician may find that he or she is actually performing few of the operations, a situation that can result in deteriorating skills.

As we consider how to maintain, even enhance, clinical skills while working in academic medicine, let us look at what is different about clinical practice in the academic medical center (AMC), how to keep your abilities up to date, and where you can learn more.

Clinical Care in the AMC

Faculty Practice Group

As an academic clinician, you will almost certainly see patients under the umbrella of a faculty practice group. The good news is that this arrangement will relieve you of the need to become involved in practice management (unless you choose to do so). The bad news is that you will give up a great deal of autonomy in regard to work hours, scheduling patients, referral options, and after-hours coverage. One of the big problems academic faculty practice groups face is helping clinicians entering academics from private practice learn how to work within the academic group constraints.

Finding Your Clinical Niche

You may want to think of some service you can provide that sets you apart. I am a member of a family medicine department, and we family physicians are the consummate generalists. However, in our department there are physicians who offer "special services" that include geriatric care, travel medicine, sports medicine, end-of-life care, complementary and alternative medicine, and a variety of office-based procedures. Another example: In our institution, a physician approaching retirement developed an interest in treating musculoskeletal problems with dimethylsulfoxide (DMSO). This physician attracted a sizable practice, including some people who came from out-of-state just for the specialized treatments. By finding a niche, this physician prolonged his clinical career and provided a service valued by his patients.

Finding a clinical niche does not mean that you must do sports medicine or acupuncture all day every day. But it does mean that you offer a service that sets you apart, may become a focus for your scholarly activities, and can generate internal referrals within your practice group.

Clinical Records

AMCs have a tradition of dysfunctional clinical records. The problems have arisen from the practice of combining clinic (outpatient) charts with voluminous hospital records. To make matters worse, these combined records tended to be stored in a central repository in the hospital, far from where they are needed when the patient visited a clinic. To overcome this inconvenience, clinics began to maintain their own separate patient-care records, containing information that did not find its way into the combined record in the hospital.

It gets worse. Faculty clinicians often take telephone calls from their academic offices, located some distance from the hospital record room and the clinic's supplementary record room. This led to the practice of maintaining "shadow charts" on private patients—informal file folders maintained by individual physicians, housed in their academic offices, sometimes containing data recorded nowhere else and available only to the individual faculty physician.

Fortunately, electronic medical records (EMRs) promise to correct these problems, with a single, easy-to-use clinical record for each patient that is available from any computer (if you have the proper password). Private practice groups and some faculty practices are already using EMRs exclusively, often with no paper records at all. Many AMCs are, like my institution, currently at the awkward transition phase of offering some data on EMR and also maintaining some paper records, but that duality will end before long.

Staying Current with Clinical Skills

Self-Assessment

Are you up to date? A good starting point is self-assessment. Are your clinical skills what they were when you entered academics? Have you kept current with advances in medicine? A good tool can be the periodic recertification examination offered by many specialties. All member boards of the American Board of Medical Specialties (ABMS), the umbrella organization for the 24 approved medical specialty boards in the United States, offer recertification programs and time-limited certificates of various durations.[1,2] Although many still use multiple-choice questions, the examinations can give some indication of where you stand with today's medical knowledge. Expect a modest decline in your score with advancing age; a sharp drop in your examination score should cause you to question your clinical abilities.

The current best method of examination uses computer-based simulations and standardized patients to assess the clinical skills of practicing physicians.[3] This type of assessment is currently used in many recertification examinations because it is more likely to mirror what happens in practice than "best choice of five possible answers" questions.

The future for all of us is the Maintenance of Certification (MOC) initiative of the ABMS, "which sets a standard requiring doctors to assess and improve the quality of their practice performance."[4] The focus of the MOC is actual enhancement of practice quality after evaluation of a physician's practice performance. As this is written, tools are being developed to permit physicians to assess their performance, compare their performance to benchmarks, and formulate quality improvement initiatives.

Educational Options Available

The options available to academic clinicians to maintain and enhance clinical performance are not much different from those obtainable by doctors in private practice. Granted, academic clinicians have the opportunity to participate in many educational seminars intended for residents and students, but the faculty member may be too busy to attend. Also, often the faculty member is the teacher who presents a lecture or a workshop on a single topic—such as chest pain or brain tumors—over and over again, a series of activities that is not expanding the teacher's broad medical knowledge very much.

It is a very good idea for academic clinicians to attend a clinical refresher course each year, especially if in a generalist specialty. Every specialty offers some sort of course, and the demand (and hence the number of courses) is growing with the increase in specialty recertification.

If your clinical work involves procedures—and today that includes most medical specialties—I suggest that you attend a hands-on procedural workshop every year or two. You may aim to improve your skills in a procedure you already perform from time to time or might learn a totally new technique. Remember that when laparoscopic abdominal surgery first became technically possible, surgeons needed to attend workshop courses to learn the new technique.

Where to Learn More

Table 5.1 tells where you can learn more about maintaining patient care skills in academic medicine. In addition, the

TABLE 5.1. Information sources about patient care in the academic medical center

---

Articles, books, and Web sites

Berg D. Advanced clinical skills and physical diagnosis. Malden MA: Blackwell, 2004.

Guyatt G, Rennie D, eds. User's guides to the medical literature; a manual for evidence-based clinical practice. Chicago: AMA Press, 2002.

Hawkins R, MacKrell GM, LaDuca T, et al. Assessment of patient management skills and clinical skills of practicing doctors using computer-based simulations and standardized patients. Med Educ 2004;39:958–968.

Healthstream: available at http://www.healthstream.com/. This company's goal is to provide learning solutions for the health care industry.

McLennan G. Is the master clinician dead? Acad Med 2001;76:617–619.

Selected organizations

American Academy on Physician and Patient: available at http://physicianpatient.org. This organization focuses on research, education, and practice in patient-physician communication.

American Board of Medical Specialties: available at http://www.abms.org. Go here to learn more about specialty certification, recertification, and Maintenance of Certification.

Association of American Medical Colleges, Group on Faculty Practice: available at http://www.aamc.org/members/gfp. An organization of leaders of academic faculty practice groups.

Society for Academic Continuing Medical Education: available at http://www.sacme.org. For individuals interested in presenting CME activities.

Society of Hospital Medicine: available at http://www.hospitalmedicine.org. An organization of hospitalist physicians, the SHMM's mission includes enhancing the delivery of health care to the patients served by hospitalists.

Medscape Web site maintains a current directory of continuing medical education opportunities listed by specialty. Go to http://www.medscape.com/cmecenterdirectory.

CLINICAL TEACHING

Educator and writer Parker J. Palmer has written: "Good teaching is an act of generosity, a whim of wanton muse, a craft that may grow with practice, and always risky business."[5] The word "doctor" comes from the Latin word *docere*, meaning "to teach." Therefore it seems logical that if I am a good doctor for my patients, I must be a good teacher. This conclusion, of course, is not exactly true. Teaching requires a different skill set than patient care, although I don't think you can be a good clinical educator *without* being a very good physician. The very worst teachers mirror the arrogance and insensitivity we see in some clinicians as they berate, humiliate, and sometimes damage students, with very little useful information shared.

About Clinical Teaching

Teaching medical students and residents may be what you came to academic medicine to do. Now would you be surprised to find that success in teaching is counterintuitive? Just as in learning to ski, you must stop doing what you want to do for safety's sake—lean into the hill—and instead do what seems "wrong:" that is, you must put your weight on the downhill ski. In teaching, our first instinct is to tell the resident or student what we know, sometimes *all* we know. But that is not the ideal teaching. The best bedside and outpatient clinic educators help the learner discover the right answers, and they do so by a series of carefully crafted questions.

Clinical teaching has some special characteristics: It describes what happens between a learner and a clinical instructor in relationship to a patient encounter, focusing either on a clinical problem affecting the patient or on the patient's response to the problem.[6] In contrast to, for example, the teaching of biology or English literature, medical education uses an apprentice model.[7] Also, because clinical teaching involves a problem-solving approach related to patients and because there is little way to predict what patients may come to the clinic or be admitted to the hospital overnight, the clinical teacher must "be prepared to discuss a diversity of medical problems without knowing what to prepare for."[8]

Characteristics of the Ideal Clinical Teacher

J. Michael Bishop, 1989 Nobel Prize in Medicine winner, writes that his three priorities in teaching are first, to inspire;

second, to challenge; and third and only third, to impart information.[9] The ideal clinical teacher inspires an enthusiasm for learning that goes beyond solving the immediate problem; this educator imparts the worth of intellectual inquiry. I believe that part of *inspiring* is acting as a role model and mentor for the learner, which Bell suggests will help us avoid being "accused of producing physicians who are superbly trained, but poorly educated."[10]

Second, good educational technique involves providing a *challenge* to the learner. In the clinical setting, this challenge classically takes the form of insisting that the student commit to a diagnosis and a plan of management before going on with discussion. Less important, but often helpful to the learner, is *sharing information* with the learner—the teaching point or "pearl" of the encounter. Sharing information can include looking up answers when unsure about the latest recommendations on a topic such as the management of unstable diabetes mellitus or metastatic prostate cancer.

Here is an example of a teaching encounter: My intern presented a 52-year-old man with a painful vesicular rash on the right side of the face, specifically in the area of the ophthalmic division of the trigeminal nerve. The intern correctly identified the rash as herpes zoster and planned to treat the patient with acyclovir—a good choice. I asked the intern if the patient had vesicles on the tip of the nose, which could be the harbinger of ophthalmic zoster; this fact was new information for the learner and represented a sharing of information.

The ideal clinical teacher has a keen awareness that "To teach is to learn twice." This short sentence, indicating that both educator and learner benefit from the teaching encounter, is attributed to Joseph Joubert, the Inspector General of Education for France who died in 1824. Ironically, Joubert wrote little and never published. His ideas lived on in his students and in a few scribbled thoughts he called *papiers de la malle* (scraps of paper). These collected thoughts were published after his death.[11]

A Model for Clinical Teaching

A widely used model of clinical teaching is called the "One-Minute Preceptor" (OMP). The model arose from a paper by Neher and colleagues, which described five "microskills" of clinical teaching.[12] Over the years, the One-Minute Preceptor has been refined and validated in a variety of teaching settings, including the clinic, hospital bedside, and—in my opinion—in small-group discussions (see the model below). When compared to traditional precepting models, the OMP has been found to shift teaching points away from generic clinical skills toward disease-specific teaching.[13] It also enhances the efficiency of the teaching encounter and improves the diagnosis of the patients' medical problems.[14] With the understanding that you may encounter various iterations of the One-Minute Preceptor, and that the teaching encounter usually takes more than 60 seconds (a 5- to 10-minute educational session is more likely), the following is a précis of the model.[15]

The One-Minute Preceptor consists of five steps:

1. **Commitment:** Begin by having the learner make a commitment: "What do you think is the diagnosis?" "Why did the patient come to the office today?" Or "What therapy should you recommend?"

2. **Support:** Seek evidence to back up the commitment made in step 1. "What are the history and physical findings that lead you to your diagnosis?" "What is the evidence for choosing the drug you recommend?"

3. **Reinforce:** Provide specific praise for insightful and well-supported commitment decisions. "Based on the historical data and physical findings you describe, I concur with your diagnosis." "Evidence-based guidelines support your management plan."

4. **Correct:** Point out any errors in the learner's facts or reasoning. "The history and physical exam findings would lead me to a different diagnosis." "I believe the current evidence now supports another management regimen."

5. **Teach:** Tell one principle that is relevant to the case, considering what you would like the learner to remember

from the encounter: "The next time you see a patient with these findings, I suggest that you think of. . . ." "Don't forget to consider the uncommon diagnosis; eventually someone will turn up with the rare disease." "When in doubt about managing a disease that is the subject of rapidly changing clinical recommendations, it is always a good idea to consult the literature."

If you think you will have a problem remembering the five steps—commitment, support, reinforce, correct, teach—try the following mnemonic that will help you recall the first letter of each word: "Clinical Specialists Really Can Teach."[15] Master this technique and you will set a high standard for your faculty colleagues teaching in the clinic, the hospital, and small-group settings.

Types of Learners

The clinician new to academics soon learns that all learners are not alike, any more than all patients are alike. As patient-care physicians, you and I might logically expect all our learners to be motivated, eager, informed, and respectful. This is, however, not the case. Be prepared to meet the following learners early in your academic medicine teaching career:

- Average Joe or Jane Learner: Although not as eager and motivated as we educators would prefer, average Joe and Jane will assimilate material presented, carry their weight in small-group discussions, and perform capably in the hospital or clinic. These learners, while not always inspiring to teach, are not a problem.
- The Needy Learner: This learner requires a lot of extra help and knows it. The needy learner also craves self-validation. Although often mute during group discussion, this learner may have a lot of questions, especially after class or by appointment in your office. He or she seldom has original ideas and leans heavily on classmates. After spending time with this learner, you will feel a little drained. In the end, the needy learner is rarely an academic standout.

■ The Competitive Learner: This learner, self-assured and headed for the top, is the opposite of the needy learner. The competitive learner can dominate a small group, but he or she is also the learner who brings in the key paper that brings new insight to a discussion. Any grade less than "honors" is likely to be challenged. Confident teachers often like the competitive learner; insecure teachers may be threatened.

■ The Solo Learner: This learner marches to his or her own drumbeat. The solo learner likes to do independent research on clinical topics but generally does not share findings with the group. The solo learner studies alone, and forgoes the benefits of collaborative learning. For the intellectually gifted learner, this method can be just fine; for those who are not intellectually gifted, being a solo learner can be a path to poor performance.

■ The Avoidant Learner: Is this person still in school? In residency? No one has seen the avoidant learner recently. The individual may be inundated with information and responsibility. Or the avoidant learner is, for one reason or another, really not interested. In a clinical setting, the avoidant learner tries hard to have as little contact as possible with preceptors. Learners with alcohol, drug, or clinical depression problems often become viewed as avoidant learners.

Respecting the Power Differential

As a newcomer to academic medicine, it is well to consider the issue of power. A faculty member—even the newly minted clinical instructor—is viewed by learners as having immense power over them. These learners believe that the faculty literally can affect their futures, largely through grades and subsequently with recommendations for residency and fellowship positions. Hence, there is an inescapable power differential, even though learners and faculty may work side by side in patient care. The best academic clinicians are aware of this differential, of the learner's perceived dependence on our approval and good will. Faculty should treat all learners with the respect they deserve and maintain professional awareness of the power they hold when dealing with learners in any setting.

Some Thoughts about Teaching Settings

You will teach in several settings. Some—the clinic and the hospital—will have patients involved. Others—the small group/seminar discussion, workshop, and lecture—will not.

Patient-Care Setting

In many instances, the "classroom" is the hospital bedside or the clinic examination room. Here teaching involves at least three persons: the learner, the teacher, and the patient. The patient must be involved in the teaching and cannot just become a "diseased organ" without a voice or respect. I am proud that some of my clinic patients have considered themselves *teaching cases* and proudly challenged generations of learners to "hear the murmur" or examine some other known physical abnormality.

In a sense, patient-care–related teaching is capricious. It is dependent on the clinical problems present in hospitalized patients or in patients who come to the clinic. I once worked with a young general internist who was a recent graduate of a good residency program in a major city. This physician had never seen a patient with pityriasis rosea; during his AMC training, patients with recent-onset skin rashes went to the emergency department, dermatology clinic, or somewhere other than his general medicine service. They certainly were not admitted to the hospital. Thus, when the young physician encountered his first patient with pityriasis rosea in practice, he failed to think of the diagnosis and instead launched into a workup looking for syphilis, psoriasis, Lyme disease, or Rocky Mountain spotted fever.

Teaching in the patient-care setting is the domain of the One-Minute Preceptor strategy. Some of the five steps can be initiated when the patient is present, but generally the encounter takes place outside the patient's room. Correcting learner errors within earshot of the patient undermines the patient's confidence, and considering a variety of diagnostic and therapeutic alternatives can mislead the patient and cause unnecessary worry.

Currently, we are seeing patient-care teaching move from the hospital to the outpatient setting. The reason is today's shorter hospital stays. Patients with many health problems that once required week-long hospital stays are now discharged in 36–48 hours. In a sense, hospitals are becoming large intensive-care units. The short interval between admission and discharge does not allow leisurely study of hospitalized patients with disease.

In the end, fundamental principles of teaching apply in the clinic and in the hospital setting. The best teachers set learning objectives and help students learn how to find answers. They also demonstrate their own clinical competence while allowing learners to assume progressively greater responsibility for decisions. In addition, they make themselves available to students and residents outside of scheduled teaching times.[16]

Small-Group Discussions

The discussion group is a favored educational method. One study seems to show that the model yields better learning than lectures. Dunnington and colleagues report that "regardless of topic or testing method, students in problem-oriented small group sessions (POSGS) tended to perform better than students in didactic lectures (DL) and that POSGS offers significant advantages over the DL in teaching surgery to third-year medical students."[17]

When all goes well, group discussion fosters problem solving, innovative thinking, integration of diverse data, and sometimes attitudinal adjustment. Participants learn communication skills, listening skills, and effective meeting behavior. For the institution, small group teaching is "resource-intensive," meaning that if 100 students sit in a lecture for an hour, only one teacher is needed, but for the same hour 10 teachers would be needed to lead 10 small groups of 10 students each.

Small-group discussion should be what it says—discussion. In a sense, group discussion is like clinical teaching because of the need to respond to the unexpected, calling for the leader to be creative and sometimes open-minded. What may be different is the amount of "expert knowledge" needed. In the patient-care setting, the academic clinician needs to have a high degree of patient-care skills; in the group-discussion setting, the facilitator can always turn the difficult question back to the group or use it as an assignment for next week.

The inexperienced faculty member may want to arrive with a PowerPoint presentation and then lecture to the 10 people in the room, fielding a few questions at the end. This wastes a valuable educational opportunity and often bores the learners. Experienced and confident small-group leaders prepare questions for discussion, sometimes have learners seek answers to some questions before the session, and then let the group participate freely in the conversation. Good small-group discussion leaders are good listeners and are not afraid of a short period of silence. They tend to facilitate discussion with open-ended questions, rather than provide answers or tell personal anecdotes.

Small-group discussion requires small groups. A minimum group may be three persons. I consider the functional maximum to be about 12 persons; above that number, most participants will not get a satisfying amount of "air time," and the avoidant and solo learners will be able to escape without participating as they should. For years, I have taught a monthly small-group seminar on headache diagnosis and management to 9–12 third-year medical students. Recently, the medical school increased the overall class size, and I now find that my typical group has 16 students. The increased size has changed the dynamics of the seminar, and I believe that its value as a learning activity has dropped a little.

Here are some useful hints when leading a small group that meets for several sessions over time:

- Start your group session exactly on time; waiting for latecomers teaches everyone to be late.
- As leader, sit in a different seat every week. This forces movement in the group and breaks up cliques.

■ Ask everyone to prepare something to bring to the session, promoting "buy-in" to the group process. Then have everyone share what he or she learned. For example, I have asked groups of students to bring in an interesting medical word origin, a clinical pearl of wisdom, or a medical aphorism. I believe that the assignments can be viewed as an enrichment activity and need not necessarily be directly related to the formal discussion topic.

■ Frame the discussion question carefully and then allow response before saying much more. Let the group shape the discussion, unless going far afield.

■ Be sure everyone gets to speak. If you have an apparently mute participant, ask this learner for an opinion. A good question is "Who hasn't spoken yet?" Permit no one to stay silent for the entire session.

■ Don't let one competitive learner dominate the discussion.

■ Think ahead to the next session and describe the "homework" assignment.

■ End the session on time.

Workshops

I consider a workshop much like a small-group discussion, except that there will be a skill learned or a task completed. A skill learned may be how to apply a forearm cast or suture a lacerated pig's foot. A task completed might be actively preparing an outline or writing a paragraph in a medical writing workshop.

Workshops may require more leader preparation than other teaching models. You need more than a few provocative questions. There must be a plan of how the time will be used. Some materials—such as casting or suturing items—may be needed.

Workshops fail when the group is too large, there aren't enough materials, or the use of time is not thoughtfully planned. Well-conceptualized and executed workshops—such as the technique of breast examination or how to perform flexible sigmoidoscopy—can be outstanding learning experiences.

Lectures

What about lectures? Didn't we spend most of our medical school hours in lectures? In his novel *Walden Two*, B. F. Skinner wrote, "The lecture is the most inefficient method of diffusing culture. It became obsolete with the invention of printing. It survives only in our universities and a few other backward institutions. . . ."[18]

Nevertheless, the lecture remains a favored form of teaching in medical school. One reason is that it is a cost-effective use of faculty time. Also, although many students learn best in small-group discussion and while the solo learner may learn best alone, some students prefer lectures and assimilate knowledge best in this setting.

All of us will, eventually, plan and deliver lectures. When the time comes to do so, begin by writing out the goals for the lecture. Then develop a concept: If lecturing about asthma to medical students, will I use the traditional format of epidemiology, pathophysiology, manifestations, diagnosis, therapy, and prevention? Or will I tell: What's new in Dx and Rx of asthma? Probably the "what's new" concept is better for practicing physicians. How about: "Ten Things You Need to Know About Asthma?" Or think of a different way to present the topic. Then expand your concept into a talk that will allow an opportunity for discussion and that does not exceed the allotted time.

Decide if you will use PowerPoint for your lecture. Almost certainly you will, as this is a handy way to share your outline with a large audience and avoid fumbling with index cards at the podium. Just be sure that your slides don't have too many words and that each phrase can be read from the back of the room.

Here are some tips to help you prepare and deliver better lectures:

■ Recognize that everyone gets a little nervous when asked to lecture. A newspaper once conducted a poll asking respondents about their greatest personal fears. The leading fear mentioned by most of those polled was public speaking, well ahead of death, which was ranked number four.[19]

■ If possible, move out from behind the lectern, so that there is nothing physically between you and the audience. A lavaliere microphone helps with this maneuver.

■ Begin by asking the audience a question that requires a verbal response or raising hands. This wakes up the audience, helps get them involved, and helps get you past your initial anxiety.

■ Use an opening humorous anecdote only if it is very pertinent, very funny, and not offensive to anyone on earth. Tell a joke only if you are really very good at joke telling.

■ Right at the start, tell the audience what you are going to tell them—the goals and the outline of the lecture. Then stick to the plan.

■ Consider using an illustrative case. The best such case is one that you can return to at different points in the lecture.

■ For every generalization you make, be sure to provide a concrete example.

■ Be sure to present and develop your points logically and in an order that makes sense.

■ From time to time, tell the audience where you are in the journey and how far from the destination.

■ End your lecture with a summary of important points to remember. Stated succinctly: Tell 'em what you told 'em.

■ Finish in time to allow some questions and discussion. Talking beyond your allotted time is rude to your audience, who are now awkwardly deciding if it is safe to leave while you are still talking, and also to the lecturer who follows you.

Evaluation and Feedback

Evaluation is an integral part of all aspects of academic medicine, including teaching. Evaluation of learners is important to assure that important content is being assimilated, that learners are able to apply information learned, and that educational goals are being met. As much as we would like to believe otherwise, evaluation remains quite subjective, including decisions as to what will be evaluated and how evaluation will occur. In addition, our current standards as to how medicine should be practiced become reflected in our evaluation of learners.

Evaluation is, of course, a two-way street, and all activities of academic clinicians are assessed by learners, peers, and supervisors. This multifaceted and ongoing evaluation process is grounded in the value system of the academic medical center and it guides who gets the rewards, as described in Chapter 3. In this chapter, however, I will focus on evaluating learners.

Fundamentally, there are two types of evaluation: Formative evaluation, sometimes called a "midcourse correction," is feedback intended to influence a change. Formative evaluation may not become part of one's permanent record. For example, during a clerkship, the teacher may note that a learner consistently keeps his head buried in the chart when talking to patients or that she that repeatedly neglects to take a family history. Those observations may be shared with the learner during formative evaluation, without being recorded on the record. Formative evaluation given orally is sometimes called feedback.

Summative evaluation, on the other hand, goes "on the record." This type of evaluation is a summary of the learner's performance on a clerkship or other educational experience. A grade of some sort may be part of a summative evaluation.

Methods of Evaluation

Evaluation takes one of two general forms: observation and objective testing.

Observation is the basis of most learner evaluation in AMCs. Whether using checklists, videotape interpretation, anecdotal recollections, or even chart review, observational evaluation is inherently subjective. It is difficult to separate the person from the behavior. Hence one must always wonder if we give higher scores to people who seem to be "like us" than to those who are not like us. Do we favor those who mirror our values and opinions? Clearly, evaluation is subject to bias, and hence whenever possible, we temper observation with something we believe is objective.

Objective testing makes us feel that our evaluations are fair and unbiased. Multiple choice testing is more-or-less objective, except that it favors the gifted test-taker—the intuitive person who can often discern the intent of the question. I once edited a book on examination questions. There were 1200 multiple-choice questions, and the book was intended as a practice exercise for those physicians taking a board certification examination. In compiling this book, I asked one author to write a chapter on test taking. The result was a series of principles to help the reader figure out questions, even when actual knowledge was limited. At the end of the chapter was a number of answer sets *without questions*; based on the rules described earlier in the chapter, there was a most-likely-correct response in each set of "answers."[20]

Self-Assessment
A sometimes-useful technique in evaluation and feedback is to elicit the learner's opinion of his or her own performance. When evaluating one's own work, one generally is more critical than an impartial observer.[21] If you ask a learner to rate his or her own performance, don't be surprised if the criticism is harsher than yours.

Principles of Academic Evaluation
The following tips may help you when you are required to evaluate learners:

- Recognize that teachers really do not like to evaluate learners. No one enjoys criticizing another, but constructive feedback is often just what the learner needs.
- If consistent with the style in your institution, use statements beginning with "I," taking ownership for the comments in the report.
- Do not inflate your evaluations. You do the learner no favor and you undermine your credibility and the credibility of your educational program. If you have 11 learners in your small group, it is highly unlikely that all performed at the "honors" level.

■ Even with my admonition about grade inflation, you should never submit an evaluation that is entirely negative. Find an achievement to praise: The student showed up for the majority of the discussion sessions. He made a good effort to meet expectations. His skills improved over the course of the clerkship. He did not injure anyone. Find something positive to say to balance, ever so slightly, the negative comments.

■ Make your evaluation performance-based. Use specific instances to support comments.

■ Do not be cute. Resist the temptation to inject a clever phrase into a written, formal evaluation.

■ Do not label. Avoid words such as "lazy," "hostile," or "difficult student," even if you believe that such an adjective is warranted. Describe behavior objectively and precisely, and allow the reader to draw conclusions.

■ If you criticize behavior in relationship to patient care, consider if you should suggest a way to change the behavior.

Be prepared to discuss your evaluation with the student after it is submitted. If your evaluation is critical and of less than "honors" quality, the student may argue that some parts of the evaluation are not really fair and that changes should be made. Perhaps some editing will be appropriate. I caution you, however, about changing letter or "honors/satisfactory" grades. If you do this once, you are marked as a faculty member who is open to grade negotiation.

Should you review your evaluation with the student before submitting to the course director? If permitted, this may not be a bad idea. It would avoid a later confrontation and possible editing of a report previously filed. The learner would know exactly what is going on the record and why. Of course, with the stellar evaluation of the gifted student, everyone is happy.

Where to Learn More

There is much more to learn about clinical teaching. Some helpful resources are found in Table 5.2. The organization

TABLE 5.2.   Information sources about clinical teaching

Articles, books and Web sites

Douglas KC, Hosokawa MC, Lawler FH. A practical guide to clinical teaching in medicine. New York: Springer, 1998.

Ende J. What if Osler were one of us? Inpatient teaching today. J Gen Int Med 2004;12(Suppl. 2):S41–S48.

Fadlon J, Pessach I, Toker A. Teaching medical students what they think they already know. Educ Health 2004;17(1):35–41.

Ramani S. Promoting the art of history taking. Med Teach 2004;26:374–376.

Ramani S, Orlander JD, Strunin L, Barber TW. Whither bedside teaching? A focus-group study of clinical teachers. Acad Med 2003;78:384–390.

Speer A, Elnicki M. Assessing the quality of teaching. Am J Med 1999;106:381–384.

Spencer J. ABC of learning and teaching in medicine. Available at http://bmj.bmjjournals.com/cgi/content/full/326/7389/591.

Sweet S. Undergraduate osteopathic medical education. J Am Osteopath Assoc 2003;103(11):507–512.

Whitman N. Notes of a medical educator. Salt Lake City: University of Utah School of Medicine, 1999.

Selected organizations*

Association for Surgical Education: available at http://www.surgicaleducation.com/.

Association of American Medical Colleges, Council of Teaching Hospitals: available at http://www.aamc.org/teachinghospitals.htm/.

Association of Directors of Medical Student Education in Psychiatry: available at http://www.admsep.org/.

Association of Teachers of Preventive Medicine: available at http://www.atpm.org/.

Society of Osteopathic Medical Educators: available at http://www.aacom.org/.

Society of Teachers of Family Medicine: available at http://www.stfm.org/.

Society for Academic Continuing Medical Education: available at http://www.sacme.org/.

Society for Academic Emergency Medicine: available at http://www.saem.org/.

Society for Education in Anesthesia: available at http://www.seahq.org/.

The Generalists in Medical Education: available at http://www.thegeneralists.org/.

*For more associations described as "Professors of. ..." and "Society of University. ..." see Table 8.2.

list includes some of the leading academic associations, in contrast to medical political organizations such as the American Medical Association. Academic association members are those with special interests in teaching and scholarship.

SCHOLARSHIP

I will remind you here that, regardless of protestations to the contrary, the key to success in the AMC is scholarship. I call this the Scholarly Imperative. If you wish to share fully in the rewards of medical academia, it is imperative that you engage in some form of scholarship. Fortunately for the academic clinician, there is much more to scholarship than randomized control trials of experimental drugs and amino acids in rat livers.

The Scholarly Imperative

Medical academia may be considered by some to be a cult of Intellectual Darwinism—with the most creative and entrepreneurial surviving, and the others often banished to obscurity, maybe even extinction. It is like a league of competitive scholarship encouraged by grant awards and cheered on by department chairs and deans. In another sense, academic scholarship is like a game played by National Basketball Association 7-foot-tall giants, functioning as teams, but not really. Each player knows that his contract is on the line every season.

The academic clinician can play in this game, without returning to school for a PhD degree and without becoming a Researcher with a capital R. The key is the expanded definition of *scholarship*.

The Expanded Definition of Scholarship

Boyer has found a way to reconcile the "teaching vs. research" debate.[22] In 1990, he proposed that there are actually four types of scholarship:

■ **The Scholarship of Discovery:** This is the research we traditionally associate with the AMC. It includes randomized, controlled studies and the like. Important goals are attaining funding support, notably from the National Institutes of Health (NIH), and publishing results in peer-reviewed journals.

■ **The Scholarship of Integration:** This scholarship develops creative insights based on merging findings from various disciplines. Here, for instance, the academic clinician might meld findings from behavioral science and pharmacology in the treatment of depression. The scholarship of integration is often documented in review articles and chapters in reference books.

■ **The Scholarship of Application:** Here we find innovative ways to bring research findings to the actual practice of medicine, the bench-to-bedside transition. A new antibiotic has been discovered; will it be effective in treating community-acquired pneumonia? Will home visits help prevent malnutrition in the elderly? What are the new methods of treating the symptoms of diabetic neuropathy, and what is the evidence for the recommendations? Scholarship of application is evidenced by publication of case reports and clinical series and by presentations at professional meeting. Today there is increasing interest in the scholarship of application. In some schools, credit is also given for clinical applications of knowledge, such as documentation of innovations in charting medical records, assessing quality of care, and monitoring clinical outcomes.

■ **The Scholarship of Teaching:** This may be the most elusive of the four types of scholarship.[23] The scholarship of teaching includes methods of communicating knowledge, skills, and problem-solving methods to learners, and the evaluation of the outcomes. Valued activities here include development of curricula, creation of teaching monographs, and construction of evaluation instruments. In addition, this type of scholarship may be documented by reports of educational methods published in scholarly journals and presented at professional meetings.

The important point is this: It is likely that your institution has considered this taxonomy and has adopted it in some way. As you present yourself for advancement in rank and in other competitive settings, do not limit your documentation to only the Scholarship of Discovery. Be prepared to present your credentials using the full expanded definition of scholarship.

Your Career Topic

In a visit to the Natural History Museum in London while writing his book *A Short History of Nearly Everything,* Bryson was introduced to an elderly scientist. "When the man departed, [my guide] said to me: "That was a very nice chap named Norman who's spent forty-two years studying one species of plant, St. John's wort. He retired in 1989, but he still comes in every week."[24]

Academic medicine adores reductionism. What does this mean to you as an academic clinician? It means that, even if you are a generalist, you must find an academic niche, both for clinical practice and scholarship; ideally these are the same topic. I call this your Career Topic. For me, as a generalist, this topic has been migraine headache. I have lectured and written on migraine. I have seen countless migraine patients. Because of my lectures and writing on headache, I became the "go-to" referral doctor in our AMC for difficult headache patient referrals. I realized then that, temperamentally, I prefer the diversity of generalism and pulled back from my meta-specialty of headaches, but I could very well have flourished as the expert in this narrow area.

My message is this: If you are to advance, to become renowned, and to be what is considered a successful academician, you must find a special niche. It is best to find this niche early in your career. Sometimes it happens almost by chance. One of my colleagues became interested in a new method of clinical breast examination; she got a grant, taught a course for practitioners and then measured the outcome. Then she got another grant, and she is well on her way to becoming a national expert in clinical breast examination. In fact, she has diverse clinical interests, but her current scholarly trajectory is headed for the stars, and it would be foolish to change course.

One reason it is important to get an early start on your Career Topic is the career cycle of scientific publications. Krumland and colleagues looked at the scientific publications of a medical school faculty.[25] They found that, over the careers of the medical school faculty studied, there were two career peaks when considering productivity as including both quantity and apparent scientific quality of publications (see Figure 5.1). The first peak, coming at a career age

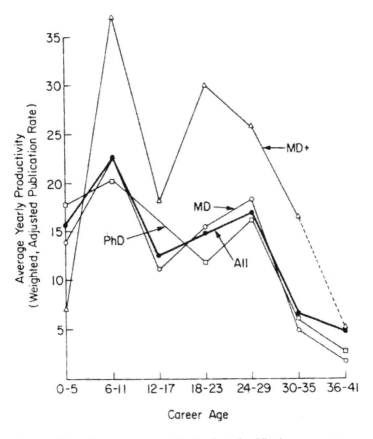

FIGURE 5.1. Average yearly, weighted, adjusted publication rate versus career age for the 4-year sample. This is a composite measure reflecting both quantity and apparent scientific quality of publications. Source: Krumland RB, Will EE, Gorry GA. Scientific publications of a medical school faculty. J Med Educ 1979;54:876–884. Used with permission.

(roughly an indication of time on faculty) of about 6–12 years, reflected "young faculty members whose relatively few publications were of high apparent quality. The second peak was for more mature faculty whose high productivity was attributable to more publications of less apparent quality."[25]

The take-home lesson is to find your Career Topic early, while you have good ideas, the energy to develop them, and the opportunity to seek a mentor to guide you along the path.

About Clinical Research

Have you ever wondered if analgesics such as acetaminophen were really any better than placebo for arthritis pain? Miceli-Richard and colleagues did more than wonder. They compared the action of acetaminophen with placebo in several hundred patients with symptomatic osteoarthritis of the knee and found the drug no more effective than the placebo (Ann Rheum Dis 2004;63:923–930).

Some astute clinician noted that the antifungal drug ketoconazole, when taken in high doses, has a testosterone-lowering effect. Subsequent clinical research was done, and now ketoconazole is used in the treatment of advanced prostate cancer (J Urol 1997;157:1204–1207).

Snyderman has written an editorial in the *Journal of the American Medical Association* (JAMA) that all young academic clinicians should read.[26] He begins with the thesis that, "The discrepancy between current medical practice and the capabilities for improvement is greater now than at any time since the early part of the last century." A major obstacle, in his opinion, is the "lack of a robust clinical research enterprise mobilized to translate basic discoveries into clinical relevance." The inevitable conclusion is that America needs to develop and nurture a new generation of clinical researchers, just the sort of "Scholarship of Application" that represents a career opportunity for the young academic clinician.

TABLE 5.3. Information sources about clinical scholarship

Articles and books
  Glassick CE, Huber MT, Maeroff G. Scholarship assessed. San Francisco: Jossey-Bass, 1997.
  Kelley WN, Randolph MA, eds. Careers in clinical research: obstacles and opportunities. Washington, DC: National Academy Press, 1994.
  Shine KI. Encouraging clinical research by physician scientists. JAMA 1998;280:1442–1444.
  Whimster WF. Biomedical research; how to plan, publish and present it. New York: Springer-Verlag, 1997.

Selected organizations
  American Federation for Medical Research (AFMR): available at http://www.afmr.org/.
  American Society for Clinical Investigation (ASCI): available at http://www.asci-jci.org/.
  North American Primary Research Group (NAPCRG): available at http://www.napcrg.org/.

Also see the list of academic organizations found in Table 5.2.

Where to Learn More About Academic Scholarship

Table 5.3 lists some sources of information about academic scholarship. You will also learn more about scholarship as you read Chapter 6, which describes selected academic scholarship skills: getting grants, planning and conducting research, and writing for publication.

REFERENCES

1. Recertification information. American Board of Plastic Surgery. Available at http://www.abplsurg.org/recertification_information.html.
2. Recertification and time-limited certification. American Board of Medical Specialties member boards. Available at http://www.abms.org/downloads/general_requirements/table6.pdf.
3. Hawkins R, MacKrell GM, LaDuca T, et al. Assessment of patient management skills and clinical skills of practicing doctors using computer-based case simulations and standardized patients. Med Educ 2004;38:958–968.
4. Horowitz SD, Miller SH, Miles PV. Board certification and physician quality. Med Educ 2004;38(1):10–17.

5. Palmer PJ. Good teaching: a matter of living the mystery. Change 1990;22(1):10–16.

6. Stritter FT, Baker RM, Shahady EJ. Clinical instruction. In: Handbook for the academic physician. McGaghie WC, Frey JJ, eds. New York: Springer-Verlag, 1986, p. 98.

7. Charney E. Pediatric education in community settings. In: Pediatric education in community settings: a manual. DeWitt TG, Roberts KB, eds. Arlington, VA: National Center for Education in Maternal and Child Health, 1996, p. 2.

8. Douglas KC, Hosokawa MC, Lawler FH. A practical guide to teaching clinical medicine. New York: Springer, 1998, p. 7.

9. Bishop JM. Infuriating tensions: science and the medical student. J Med Educ 1984;59(2):91–102.

10. Bell RM. Presidential address. Am J Surg 1987;154:465–469.

11. Joseph Joubert. New Advent. Available at http://www.newadvent.org/cathen/08526a.htm.

12. Neher JO, Gordon KC, Meyer B, Stevens N. A five-step "microskills" model of clinical teaching. J Am Board Fam Pract 1992;5:419–424.

13. Irby DM, Aagaard E, Teherani A. Teaching points identified by preceptors observing one-minute preceptor and traditional preceptor encounters. Acad Med 2004;79:50–55.

14. Aagaard E, Teherani A, Irby DM. Effectiveness of the one-minute preceptor model for diagnosing the patient and learner: proof of concept. Acad Med 2004;79:42–49.

15. Practical preceptorship: an effective and efficient teaching model for the on-the-go clinical preceptor. Available at http://wtce.utb/cehealth/Preceptor/one.htm.

16. McGee SR, Irby DM. Teaching in outpatient clinic. J Gen Intern Med 1997:12 (Suppl. 2):S34–S39.

17. Dunnington G, Witzke D, Rubeck R, Beck A, Mohr J, Putnam C. A comparison of the teaching effectiveness of the didactic lecture and the problem-oriented small group session: a prospective study. Surgery 1987;102:291–296.

18. Skinner BF. Walden two. New York: Macmillan, 1948.

19. McGaghie WC, Frey JJ. Handbook for the academic physician. New York: Springer-Verlag, 1986, p. 305.

20. Goodenough GK. Test-taking techniques. In: Taylor's family medicine review. Taylor RB, ed. New York: Springer-Verlag, 1999, pp. 1–7.

21. Windish DM, Knight AM, Wright SM. Clinician-teachers' self-assessments versus learners' perceptions. J Gen Intern Med 2004;19:554–557.

22. Boyer EL. Scholarship reconsidered: priorities of the professoriate. Princeton, NJ: Carnegie Foundation for the Advancement of Teaching, 1990.
23. Glassick CE. Boyer's expanded definitions of scholarship, the standards for assessing scholarship, and the elusiveness of the scholarship of teaching. Acad Med 2000;75:877–880.
24. Bryson B. A short history of nearly everything. New York: Basis Books, 2003.
25. Krumland RB, Will EE, Gorry GA. Scientific publications of a medical school faculty. J Med Educ 1979;54:876–884.
26. Snyderman R. The clinical researcher—an "emerging species." JAMA 2004;291:882–883.

6

Advanced Academic Skills: Doing Research, Getting Grants, and Writing for Publication

In Chapter 5, I described some important facts you need to know about basic academic skills: clinical care, teaching, and scholarship. I cautioned that I definitely was not telling everything you need to know, and I supplied lists of sources for further study. Here in Chapter 6, I am going to do the same—describe key aspects of advanced academic skills, with no attempt to *cover it all*. I have selected three advanced academic skills for this chapter: research, notably how to write a research protocol; the process of getting a grant; and the fundamentals of writing for professional publication.

RESEARCH

Many—and, I hope, most—academic clinicians will conduct clinical research, which has been defined as "a component of medical and health research intended to produce knowledge valuable for understanding human disease, preventing and treating illness, and promoting health."[1] The astute reader will recognize these issues as just what we do in clinical practice, including topics such as disease mechanisms, health maintenance, therapeutic interventions, and outcomes of various health services.

With this introduction, I could take the discussion in many directions. I will present two areas that I consider of key importance: these are the research question and the investigative plan, written as the research protocol.

The Research Question

I cannot overstate the value and importance of a well-conceived research question. The question is valuable because, if properly studied, it might change how medicine is practiced, if only just a little. Also, a well conceived, conducted, and reported study can launch an entire career. This happened to several researchers some 50+ years ago who asked if cigarette smoking just might lead to lung cancer later in life; some of these investigators went on to work on variations of this topic throughout long careers. The research question is important, because it will be the basis of the study, and if the question is poorly constructed or otherwise flawed, the entire research project will be in jeopardy.

The query may be framed as a formal hypothesis or as a simple question. As an example, I will continue the question of cigarette smoking and lung cancer. A hypothesis would be "Cigarette smoking causes a subsequent increase in the incidence of lung cancer in smokers when compared with non-smokers." Sometimes investigators prefer a null hypothesis, to be proved or disproved by the data: "Cigarette smoking does not cause a subsequent increase in the incidence of lung cancer." Sometimes we see a statement telling the objective of the study: "To assess whether cigarette smoking causes a subsequent increase in the incidence of lung cancer." Or the issue may be simply stated as a research question: "Does cigarette smoking cause a subsequent increase in the incidence of lung cancer?"

There is no shortage of researchable hypotheses that arise in daily practice or perhaps from reading the medical literature. You need only to keep your mind tuned to the unanswered question you encounter when seeing patients. Here are some current researchable issues:

- Does daily consumption of antibiotics decrease the risk of Alzheimer's disease?
- How often should adult women receive clinical breast examinations?
- Does a switch in health plans adversely affect health care outcomes?

- Is live influenza virus vaccine safe for children with asthma?
- Does drinking red wine help protect patients against cancer?
- Might phosphodiesterase inhibitors, such as sildenafil (Viagra) have a role in treating pulmonary vascular disease?
- Do multivitamin supplements affect human immunodeficiency virus (HIV) disease progression and mortality?
- Might antihypertensive drugs help reduce adverse cardiovascular events in patients with coronary artery disease and normal blood pressure?

Of course, once you discover a research question that sparks your interest, you will begin to study what is already known about the topic, using a literature search on MEDLINE (at PubMed.com) or another favorite site. You will think about how you will answer the question, which will raise issues such as the age groups to be studied, how many subjects will be needed, exactly what you will do to the subjects, what data you will collect, how you will analyze the data, and how you will organize the data once it is analyzed.

At this point, I urge that you enlist at least two other persons to participate in the project. One of these persons should be someone who knows more about research methods than you do. Ideally, this person will be a senior researcher who will help you refine your question, plan the project, and act as a research mentor, at least for the duration of your study. Another person will be someone who understands statistics. The statistical expert may be the most difficult to find, but you should recruit this person to the team early. With early full membership on the team, the statistician can help you avoid common methodologic and statistical pitfalls. The worst approach of all is to collect a large pile of data and then drop it on the desk of a statistician who had no prior participation in the research project. Other persons may join the team as well, each bringing some area of special expertise.

Your next step, together with your assembled research team, is to write a research protocol. Do not even think of starting a research project without completing this vital planning exercise. In fact, you probably couldn't skip the step even if you wished, because your institutional review board (IRB) will insist on reviewing the protocol as a condition of approval.

Writing a Research Protocol

No sports team would ever begin an important contest without a "game plan." The research protocol is the game plan for your project. It tells what you hope to accomplish and how you will get it done. It also imposes a discipline, requiring you and your team to anticipate every step of the project before the first subject is recruited.

For handy reference, Table 6.1 tells the basic elements of a research protocol, with some comments on the various topics to be covered.

I like to think of a research protocol as the framework for the paper that will report the study's findings. To this end, I think that a good early exercise is to prepare the format for tables that will go in the final report to be submitted for publication. Let us, for example, think about a study looking at the safety of giving live influenza virus vaccine to children with asthma. In the final report, you may have a table describing subjects by age, gender, ethnicity, and other characteristics. You might then have a table of adverse outcomes—asthma attacks, bronchitis, or pneumonia in patients who did and did not receive the vaccine. Then you may have another table showing the incidence of influenza, with and without complications, in both the study group who received the vaccine and those who did not. In this way, the tables are already conceptualized; they await only the data from the study.

The research protocol will be submitted to the IRB and also to the funding agency (aka grantor) if grant support is sought. You should spend a lot of time and energy developing the protocol, not only because it will determine if you get IRB approval and grant funding, but also because this is the plan you will follow in the months to come.

TABLE 6.1. Basic elements of a research protocol

Study name: The title of project
Primary investigator (PI) and co-investigators
Overview: I urge that you provide a very short overview, even if not
    requested on RFP outline.
Background and rationale
  What is the problem you are trying to solve?
  What prior work has been done?
  What is your research question or hypothesis?
Method
  What is your study design: Will you use a randomized trial, case control,
    cohort study, or other type of design?
  Who will be the study subjects: Who is included and who isn't, and why?
    How did you decide on this number of subjects? How will subjects be
    recruited?
  What you will do to the study subjects?
  How you plan to analyze the data? Tell specific statistical studies to be
    used.
What are possible benefits to the individual subjects?
What are risks to the subjects, and what have you done to minimize risks?
Compensation of subjects: Will study subjects be paid and, if so, how much
    and when?
Informed consent: Include a copy of the consent document.
Institutional approvals: Action of the institutional review board
Letters of agreement from other departments or clinics
Ethical issues, including confidentiality
Budget and funding
Other issues: HIPAA, data storage, etc.
Curriculum vitae of the PI and all co-investigators: These are often appended
    to the research protocol.

HIPAA, The Health Insurance Portability and Accountability Act of 1996, RFP, request for proposal.

What Makes a Good Research Protocol

The best research protocols have some characteristics in common:

■ Early overview: Begin with a brief summary of the project.

■ Logical progression of ideas: Use the outline in Table 6.1 to lead the reader, point by point, to a clear understanding of what you plan to do and how you will do it.

- Carefully constructed headings: The research protocol is really an essay. Use headings to announce how ideas are grouped.
- Clear prose: Make the document easy to read.
- Completeness: Anticipate the question a reader might have, and try to provide an answer.

Common Problems in Research Protocols

This section describes mistakes we make in research planning. Some of the common ones are:

- Vague research question: Often this means the question is too broad and needs to be focused.
- Flawed research design: Do not select a study type that will not answer the question.
- Too many research questions: I think a study can answer up to three related research questions. More than that suggests a lack of focus. I once encountered data from a study that had listed 57 research questions. In preparing a paper, the investigators struggled to find just a few questions whose answers had statistical significance. They never succeeded in writing a publishable paper.
- Inadequate number of subjects to answer the question: This is a failure of early statistical reckoning and can be a fatal flaw in the study. Do not count on the IRB to alert you to this problem, which poses no risk to subjects.
- Inappropriate plan for statistical analysis: The statistician is planning to use the wrong tests to look at the data.
- Poorly written consent form: Your IRB will send the consent form back for rewriting if not comprehensive and legally sound.

Some Thoughts About Clinical Research

Here are some random musings about clinical research and the academic clinician.

Learn to Be a Good Principal Investigator

The principal investigator (PI) is the team leader, not unlike a chief executive officer (CEO) of a company, and is usually the person who developed and championed the research question. In addition to having research skills appropriate for the study, this individual should have administrative abilities, commitment, flexibility, and integrity. A PI needs to be able to delegate without abdicating. If things go wrong in a research project, the PI must take the blame.

Do Not Try to Do Too Much Too Early in Your Career

One common error of the neophyte researcher is planning a project that is too ambitious for one's skills or for the resources available. If you enlist a seasoned researcher for the team, a good early question to ask this veteran is, "Am I (or are we) trying to do too much in this study? Does the focus need to be limited?" For a beginning researcher with a researchable question, a pilot study is a good way to field-test the idea. A pilot study, of very limited scope, can often be internally funded by the department chair, with the understanding that success with the pilot effort should lead to a larger project that is eligible for external grant funding.

Learn Some Research Design Models and Elementary Statistical Methods

I am a strong advocate of including the statistical expert as a full member of the research team. You lose nothing and can learn a lot. With that said, I urge the new researcher to learn some elementary research models and basic statistics. For example, you should understand the difference between quantitative and qualitative research. Learn the distinctions between case control and cohort studies and randomized clinical trials. Know the statistical meaning of the word significance (see the Glossary). Get to know the concepts of probability (P), confidence intervals, and analysis of variance. You don't need to know how to perform the calculations, but you should know what the statistician is describing.

Table 6.2 lists selected books on medical statistics.

Avoid Recreational Data Collection

Do not collect data you do not need. When constructing a questionnaire, there is a compelling temptation to seek data

TABLE 6.2. Selected books on medical statistics

Altman DG. Practical statistics for medical research. London: Chapman and Hall, 1991.

Bland M. An introduction to medical statistics, 3rd ed. New York: Oxford, 2000.

Daniel WE. Biostatistics: a foundation for analysis in the health sciences. New York: Wiley, 2004.

Glatz SA. Primer of biostatistics, 5th ed. New York: McGraw-Hill, 2002.

Kirkwood B, Sterne J. Essential medical statistics, 2nd ed. New York: Blackwell, 2003.

Le CT. Introductory biostatistics. New York: Wiley Interscience, 2003.

Petrie A, Sabin C. Medical statistics at a glance. New York: Blackwell, 2005.

Riegelman RK. Studying a study and testing a test, 5th ed. Philadelphia: Lippincott, Williams & Wilkins, 2005.

just because the findings might be interesting. Do not do this. Collect only data that will help to answer your research question(s). Recreational accumulation of data can lead to data mining—the nefarious practice of sifting through a pile of research figures in a retrospective search for a nugget of data that might have statistical significance.

Meet Regularly with Your Team

Plan to meet with your research team every 2–4 weeks, vowing to continue meetings until the final paper is published. The meetings will keep momentum going, and each time the group gets together can be an opportunity for the new researcher to learn. Be sure to include everyone involved in the study, which may be the research assistants, perhaps the department grants budget coordinator, and all co-authors, including your statistician.

At the regular team meetings, don't forget to talk about the eventual report of your paper. Plan what will be included, conceptualize your tables as discussed above, and decide the order of authorship. Select your *target journal*—where you hope your paper will be published. Also construct a list of subsequent choices, just in case your paper is rejected by your first-choice target journal.

Where to Learn More About Clinical Research and Research Protocols

In Table 6.3 you will find sources where you can learn more about clinical research and research protocols.

As I near the end this section on research, I want to share a quote from Hoff: "When I finished medical school, I did not intend to do research as part of my life in surgery. That all changed when I met a mentor who inspired me during my training days. I had some protected time, assembled

TABLE 6.3. Information sources about clinical research and research protocols

Articles and books
Batavia M. Clinical research for health professionals: a user-friendly guide. New York: Elsiever, 2000.
Campbell EG, Weissman JS, Moy E, et al. Status of clinical research in academic health centers. JAMA 2001;286:800–806.
Friedman LM, DeMets DL, Furbert CD. Fundamentals of clinical trials. New York: Springer-Verlag, 1998.
Good PI. A manager's guide to the design and conduct of clinical trials. Philadelphia: Wiley, 2002.
Hulley SB, Cummings SR, Browner WS, Grady D, Hearst N. Designing clinical research: an epidemiological approach. Philadelphia: Lippincott Williams & Wilkins, 2000.
Kotchen TA, Lindquist T, Malik K, Ehrenfeld E. NIH peer review of grant applications for clinical research. JAMA 2004:291:836–843.
Nathan DG, Wilson JD. Clinical research and the NIH: a report card. N Engl J Med 2004;349:1860–1865.
Whimster WF. Biomedical research: how to plan, publish and present it. New York: Springer-Verlag, 1997.

Web sites
ClinicalTrials.gov is a service of the National Institutes of Health developed by the National Library of Medicine. Available at http://www.clinicaltrials.gov/.

Selected organizations
The American Society for Clinical Investigation: available at http://www.ascijci.org/.
National Institutes of Health (NIH)
9000 Rockville Pike
Bethesda, MD 20892
http://www.nih.gov

space and equipment, developed a hypothesis, and went to it. I'll never forget my first experiment and publication. Frankly, it was my best."[2]

As you learn more about research, plan to learn more research management skills. By this I mean how to construct research budgets and how to manage research funds. And how do you get research funds? By getting grants.

GETTING GRANTS

Eventually, you will require funding for your research, and you will then need to get a grant. Fortunately, there is a lot of money available: In 2002, $150 billion in grant funding came from the federal marketplace and $241 billion of private money was donated to nonprofit organizations as tax-deductible gifts, much of which is available as grant funding.[3] Although this amount of funding could easily cover your salary and mine for many years, getting access to the money is challenging.

Grant-getting in the United States uses a "tournament" model that involves competition, recruitment of star players, and both winners and losers.[4] When you finish this section of the chapter, I think you will have a clearer understanding of this metaphor.

The World of Grants

To begin at ground level, there are two major funding sources: government and private. Government grants may be federal, state, or local. Private grant funding sources include foundations, corporations, or professional associations.

Government Grants

State and local grant funding agencies are often politically grounded, and grants may be awarded as contracts that advance favored agendas such as care of the homeless rather than based on competition for the best proposal. If you or your department has a contact in state, county, or city government, you may have a chance of receiving state/local funding for a project. An example of such a project might be a needed statewide survey of the impact of high professional liability rates on procedure-oriented specialists. Or county leaders might need a survey of physicians as they assess the need for more or less hospital beds in the future. If offered such a contract, you must consider your need for salary support as well as the direction this might take your personal research agenda.

Federal government grants are usually competitive in nature. In deciding whether or not you are the winner in the grant "tournament," agencies will consider both the merits of the project and who is making the proposal. The research track record of the investigator and the institution influences funding decisions.

There are a number of granting agencies in the federal government, offering grants of various types. For example, there are primary care training grants available through the Bureau of Health Professions of the Health Resources and Services Administration (HRSA). For the academic clinician, the important funding source is the NIH. I urge you to learn about NIH grants and funding early in your career. A good beginning Web site is The NIH Guide to Grants and Contracts, available at http://www.grants.nih.gov/grants/guide/index.html.

Because the NIH is the source of so many grant opportunities, its policies and attitudes are especially important to the academic clinician who aspires to do NIH-funded clinical research. According to Kotchen and colleagues, "A perception exists among clinical investigators that the NIH peer review process may discriminate against clinical research." With that as a background, the authors of the report studied outcomes of grant applications submitted to the NIH by MDs versus non-MDs and those involving human subjects versus those that did not. They concluded: "Although physicians compete favorably in the peer review process, review outcomes are modestly less favorable for grant applications for clinical research than for laboratory research."[5]

Table 6.4 lists selected grant databases. The sites here may include both government and private funding opportunities.

TABLE 6.4. Selected grant databases

Agency for Healthcare Research and Quality (AHRQ) Grants On-Line
Database (GOLD). Available at http://www.GOLD@ahrq.gov/.

Community of Science (COS): A comprehensive source of funding
information that lists more than 400,000 possibilities. Available at
http://www.cos.com/.

CRISP (Computer Retrieval of Information on Scientific Projects): Provides
access to information on NIH funded projects. Available at
http://www.crisp.cit.nih.gov/.

Federal Register: available at http://www.gpoaccess.gov/fr/index.html/.

Grants.gov: A portal to search for federal grants in diverse areas. Available at
http://www.grants.gov/.

Health Resources and Services Administration (HRSA): available at
http://www.hrsa/gov/.

National Institutes of Health, Office of Extramural Research home page: Go
here to hunt for NIH medical and behavioral research grant policies,
guidelines, and funding opportunities. Available at
http://www.grants.nih.gov/grants/oer.htm/.

Private Grant Sources

Foundations, corporations, and professional societies can be a rich source of grant support and are a good place for the new faculty member to get started. There are independent foundations, such as the Northwest Health Foundation, and company foundations, such as the Robert Wood Johnson Foundation, and family foundations, such as the Ford Family Foundation. Almost any major organ or chronic disease you can name has a foundation; examples include the American Heart Association, the American Lung Association, The National Stroke Association, the American Cancer Society, and the American Diabetes Association. Funding for research projects may also be available from your specialty society, which may have its own foundation. A good general source of information about foundations is The Foundation Center, available online at http://www.fdncenter.org/.

If you are considering sending a grant proposal to a private or corporate foundation in your state, I urge that you contact your academic medical center (AMC) grant office. That office is charged to coordinate grant requests submitted to various agencies, especially those that are "local."

Their reason is as follows: The institution looks foolish if a local foundation receives several proposals from your institution, with one investigator not even aware of the other's submission. Even worse, your heart-warming grant award of $10,000 today may be blamed for a later rejection of a million-dollar proposal if the grantor chooses to make only one award to a single institution.

Another type of private grant funding is related to research conducted by pharmaceutical companies or corporations making medical or surgical equipment. One of the big surprises of young faculty members may be the amount of corporate research in AMCs. Such research might be part of a larger collaborative study with you as a listed co-investigator. It is much more likely, however, that your role will be to submit research data, based on a company-generated protocol that is being used in a number of institutions. You may have no control over what goes in the final paper and, in fact, are unlikely to see your name in print when the results are published in the medical literature. Of course, without being listed as a co-author on a published report, the effort is valueless when you become a candidate for promotion. "Then why do this research?" you ask. The answer is money, and the monetary rewards for providing pharmaceutical research services are quite high. Many medical school departments and divisions depend heavily on this income to support the salaries of faculty and staff.

Key Concepts in Grant-Getting

Here I will present some generalities that apply to various types of grant proposals. A noteworthy exception to what follows is pharmaceutical company research, in which you simply agree to abide by the terms of their contract offer or else decline to participate.

The Request for Proposal

Most grant awards begin with a Request for Proposal. The RFP is an invitation by a granting agency—government or private—to submit an application. There will be a description of the type of projects that will be considered, specific instructions, a cap on the amount that may be requested, and a submission deadline. As a hypothetical example, the American Diabetes Association might seek proposals that study the impact of type 2 diabetes on other family members in a population of Native Americans, with a maximum award of $100,000 over 3 years, and a deadline for submission about 4 months in the future.

Study the RFP carefully before taking the fateful step of beginning to outline a grant project. Be very sure that your proposed project fits exactly with what the funding agency is seeking; in the hypothetical study above, writing a proposal examining the impact on a Native American family of having a type 2 diabetic *alcoholic* in the household will probably be a waste of time.

The Program Officer

Most federal and private grant funding agencies will have a designated program officer (aka project officer) for each grant solicitation. This person is a very valuable contact. I advise early contact by telephone. A face-to-face meeting is even better. Be ready to give a brief description of your project. Then ask open-ended questions:

- How well do you think my ideas matched the intent of the proposal?
- What might be the problems with the idea?
- What else would you suggest be included?
- What would you do differently? Do you see a fatal flaw in the project design?
- What other suggestions would you have?
- What else should I know?

The program officer is likely to know a great deal about the project and the agency. It is his or her job to help you present the best proposal possible. Consult the program officer often as you work on your proposal.

A word of caution is appropriate: Do not call the program officer with foolish questions that are readily answered in the RFP or on the grantor's Web site. Also, don't call to ask questions such as, "What types of proposals are likely to be funded this year?" Be sure your questions are thoughtful and carefully constructed.

The Letter of Intent

Many foundations request a letter of intent briefly describing your project. Some federal and state funding sources are adopting this concept, and you may see the terms "proposal concept paper" or "white paper." This concise overview of your idea allows both the funding source and you to decide early if more effort is warranted. If a letter of intent is requested, think your project through carefully, pay attention to the length of letter requested (1 page, 2 pages, or some other length), and be sure to answer all questions included in the instructions.

If you are provided no prescribed format for a letter of intent or proposal concept paper, use the following as topics for the paragraphs in your letter:

- Executive summary: This is a two- or three-sentence overview of your idea and why the project is appropriate for the agency you are contacting.
- Significance of the project: Tell the problem you intend to address.
- Solution to the problem: Tell how you will address the problem and how your approach is different from others.
- Request for funds: Describe why you will need money to complete the project, with a brief overview of how funds will be used.
- A sentence thanking the potential grantor for considering your proposal, followed by your signature and full contact information.

I like letters of intent, because they provide a preview of potential success, without the full effort of preparing a long grant proposal. With that said, however, I would not submit a letter of intent without having had a conversation with the program officer.

The Budget

Some say that this is the second task, right after deciding on the concept for your proposal. The budget is certainly important. Asking for too much may sink your proposal; requesting and getting a too-small grant can cause you to be underfunded. Whatever you put in your budget, be sure to justify every item in your application. If you ask for travel funds, tell why travel is needed to make your project a success. If you request money for photocopying or postage, describe what you plan to copy and mail. Also, you must master the somewhat arcane terms used in grant budgets, including direct and indirect costs, the latter now called (at the NIH) "facilities and administrative costs," and TBA, which stands for "to be added" and may refer to faculty, staff or equipment—all dependent on successful funding.

A Title for Your Project

In the end, your proposal will be presented to a review committee who will pass judgment on its merits. I am an advocate of making the topic and the outline of the project easy to remember. Sometimes the key is a catchy acronym. An example is the recently published study "The Long-term Outcomes of Sibutramine Effectiveness on Weight Study," cunningly called the LOSE Study. (Managed Care 2004;10:369–376). "The Trial of Atorvastatin in Rheumatoid Arthritis" became the TARA Study, which brings to mind the home of Rhett Butler in *Gone With The Wind*. (Lancet 2004;363:2015–2021).

A few years ago, our department submitted a federal training grant to support a 3-year program to teach our residents about advocacy (for their patients), cultural competence, and ethical issues in medicine. It became the ACE program; the acronym made little sense in an academic setting, but the three-letter word represented a memory device to help the review committee recall the three main components of the project. The project was, in fact, approved and funded.

Another grant proposal consisting of what was, frankly, a jumble of unrelated projects was approved and funded in part, I believe, because we linked them together with the memorable title, "The New Physician's Black Bag for the 21st Century."

The Grant Proposal

A good idea for a project is important as is early contact with the program office, but success ultimately depends on a professionally prepared grant proposal. Table 6.5 tells basic components of a grant proposal. Some of these items are similar to the research protocol, but some are not, because grant proposals may describe projects other than research. If in doubt about adding and discussing a topic, I suggest including the information.

Basic Writing Principles That Apply to Grant Proposals

Fundamentally, a grant proposal is a written request for money. Hence, the writing of the document is important. The following are a few principles that apply to grant proposals of all types:

- Tell your idea early in the proposal. Do not make the reader wade through three pages of "rationale" and "obstacles to be overcome" before finding the project overview on page four.

TABLE 6.5.   Basic outline of a grant proposal

Executive summary (abstract): Briefly describe the proposal
Overview of institution: Describe your institution and project team
Background: The problem and rationale for what you plan, typically based on
     a literature review or preliminary studies
Project objectives: Your hypothesis or the aim of the project
Project method: What do you plan to do?
   Subjects, methods and analysis needed for the research project (see Table
     6.1)
   OR
   The proposed educational program or other activity
Evaluation: If appropriate, tell how you will evaluate the outcome
Timeline: This should match the duration of funding described in the RFP
Budget and budget justification
Plans for future funding
Other items
   Support letters
   Affiliation agreements
   Biographical summaries of investigators

■ Use the language in the RFP. If the RFP states that the foundation seeks grant proposals to "determine ways to improve the nutritional status of homeless women in large cities," you should use exactly that language to describe your project. You will also need to determine what is meant by "nutritional status," "homeless," "large cities," and even "women." Are 12-year-old homeless females "women?"

■ Choose your project description carefully, and then use the same words in the same manner over and over. This assures that, after reading the document, the reviewer will recall the key words. Thus, in the ACE program described above, I used the words *advocacy*, *cultural competence*, and *ethical issues in medicine* over and over, in exactly the same way each time.

■ Make the document visually interesting. The reviewer will probably receive a number of grants to read, and you want to capture his or her attention. Try to avoid using very long paragraphs. Use tables to present data, when possible. If you see a section of prose extending to several pages, consider inserting headings to break up the long string of sentences. Notice on this page that I have used bullet points to avoid large blocks of prose.

■ The document should use the font and margin size recommended in the RFP. If none is recommended, use 12-point font. Margins should be 1 inch or more on sides, top, and bottom. Don't try to gain a few more words by crowding your pages.

■ Document assertions with data and sources. Cite the literature if appropriate, but don't let your grant proposal become a literature review with 90 citations.

■ Start early and finish early. I like to begin projects early and finish them well ahead of deadlines. I hate last-minute, frantic rushes. Your institutional research services department—which must read and approve your project before it can be submitted—probably dislikes last-minute problems even more than I do.

Grant deadlines for various agencies come in cycles, and all grants must be vetted by your institutional office of research services (or some office with a similar title). Hence, if you have a grant headed for the NIH, it is likely that there are a number of other grants from other departments at your AMC that have the same deadline. For this reason, it is best to be at the head of the line by completing your proposal early. A late submission will not get the attention from the offices of research services that it deserves, a problem that becomes even worse if there is an issue with your grant.

Grant Review

Your grant proposal has been approved by your department chair and the institutional research services office. The prospective grantor has received it. Next it goes to a review panel. In a typical grant review panel, all reviewers will read your grant, while one of the reviewers will be selected to present it to the group. What are the implications of this method?

First, be sure that your proposal is appropriately titled in a way that accurately describes the project and that the reader can recall a day later. The title of the proposal is the most-read part of a grant proposal.

Next most read is the executive summary. The reviewer who presents your project to the review panel is likely to begin his or her presentation here, and this paragraph is likely to be read in front of the others around the table. Try to tell the readers your concept, the key words, and the framework you will use throughout the proposal.

In various grant review settings there will be a "score," based on the total or the average of scores submitted by the reviewers present. The scores of all grants become a continuum when it comes to deciding funding. What you will eventually hear is that your proposal is

- Approved without modification to the project or budget. Congratulations!
- Approved with modification to the project and/or budget. This is usually also considered good news.
- Approved but not funded. Your grant received a good score, but the agency ran out of money as they funded grants with even higher scores.
- Rejected, meaning that your proposal's score fell below the level needed for approval and funding.

Whatever the outcome, thank the program officer for the effort and include in your letter your appreciation for the hard work of the reviewers. If your proposal was rejected or approved but not funded, you should request a copy of the reviewers' written comments, which can guide your decision as to whether or not to resubmit the grant in the next submission cycle. If you do decide to resubmit, the reviewers' comments will be paramount as you modify the proposal.

As you read the reviewers' comments, you might find a remarkable diversity of opinion among members of the panel. You might even conclude that one or two members of the review panel did not understand the proposal, if they read it at all. If this is the case, keep this opinion to yourself, and do not write an angry letter to the grantor. Recognize that, although review panel members are selected based on expertise, there may be considerable differences in their individual knowledge of your project topic.

As you consider modifying and resubmitting the proposal in the next cycle, ask the program officer for any suggestions that might be helpful. Does the program officer think you might have a reasonable chance of acceptance if you resubmit? Is there any part of the grant proposal that the program officer thinks especially merits change? Perhaps there is a problem that was not covered in the reviewers' comments.

To learn more about the NIH review process, go to "What Happens to Your Grant Application" at http://www.csr. nih.gov/Welcome/Grant_Application_print.htm/.

Thoughts About Getting Grants

Grantsmanship

Being a well-funded grant writer is one of academia's most valued skills. It can be especially useful because many research grants can be moved from one institution to another; they follow the principal investigator, who may actually move an entire research team. In the academic world, this is powerful.

You can learn to be a skilled grantsman or -woman by pyramiding your experience. Begin by joining a research team of people more experienced than you and be willing to do the "grunt" work of organizing boilerplate, getting letters of support, and writing budget justifications. Do whatever is needed to be a team member, learn the process, and be a co-investigator on the project. Your next step is to plan your own project, organize your own research or project team, and write a grant in which you are the principal investigator.

It is also helpful to volunteer to serve on your AMC's IRB, which can be an eye-opening introduction to the many types of grant proposals considered.

After you, as PI, have submitted a grant or two and have befriended a program officer, ask the program officer how you can become a member of a grant review panel. Serving on a national review panel is highly valuable experience because you get to see the grants that others have written and learn why some succeed and some are rejected. In addition, during the review process you will spend time with leaders in your field from across the country.

Common Errors in Grant Writing

Beginning grant writers make some classic errors; experienced academicians also sometimes make missteps:

- Ignoring the instructions. When agencies have a surplus of grant applications, the first cut may be those who did not follow instructions precisely. Here is an example that is extreme, but true. In 2003, a drug-and-alcohol treatment center in Oregon had two grants rejected by a federal agency because of the width of page margins. The center had submitted funding requests totaling $703,000 but "missed out because the application margins were two-tenths of an inch too small."[6]

- Failing to recognize signals in the RFP. If the RFP seems somehow peculiar, as though one needs to have very special attributes in order to carry out the project, it is just possible that it is "wired." This means that some institution already has an inside track, and your proposal will fight an uphill battle. One way to learn if a project is wired is to ask the program officer if some institution helped write the RFP.

■ Not listening carefully to the program officer. You have just described your idea to the program officer, who replies, "What you are describing is not exactly what we usually fund." Of course, you can ignore this comment, spend weeks preparing a grant application, and receive sympathetic reviewer comments ("I wish we could have approved this well-written proposal, but. . . .") along with your rejection notice.

■ Building a fatal flaw into the proposal. One example is targeting the wrong population. I once sat in a review panel for HRSA training grants. These specific grants involved training medical students and residents. One of the most comprehensive and articulate grants we considered during the 2-day meeting involved a longitudinal educational program in an integrated continuum from college through residency. But the grant program was only for medical students and residents, not college students. We turned to the program officer, who stated that this grant could not qualify for funding. Fatal flaw. Next grant.

■ Submitting to the wrong agency. Some grantors fund research; some fund education and training. Do not waste your time by mixing these up. If you intend to combine research and training in a grant, discuss this early with the program officer.

■ Overestimating your capability. Grantors always consider if the PI has the experience and resources to get the job done. Begin with modest achievable projects with reasonable budgets. Then, after a few successes, think about more ambitious projects with larger budgets. Eventually, you may qualify to write the grant for the *big project*, but this must be earned by a track record of earlier successes. A step-by-step, patient approach offers the best chance of being a winner in the tournament of grants.

Where to Learn More About Getting Grants

There is much more to learn about getting grants. Table 6.6 has some suggestions for further study.

TABLE 6.6. Information sources about grant seeking

Articles and books

Bauer DG. The "how to" grants manual: successful grant seeking techniques for obtaining public and private grants, 5th ed. Westport, CT: Praeger, 2003.

Carlson M. Winning grants: step by step, 2nd ed. San Francisco: Jossey-Bass, 2002.

Kotchen TA, Lindquist T, Malik K, Ehrenfeld E. NIH peer review of grant applications for clinical research. JAMA 2004;291:836–843.

Nathan DG. Careers in translational clinical research—historical perspectives, future challenges. JAMA 2002;287:2424–2427.

Ogden TE, Goldberg IA. Research proposals: a guide to success. New York: Raven Press, 1995.

Reif-Lehrer L. Grant application writer's handbook. Boston: Jones & Bartlett, 2005.

Yang OO. Guide to effective grant writing. New York: Kluwer Academic/Plenum Publishers; 2005.

Web sites

Developing and writing grant proposals. Catalog of Federal Domestic assistance. U.S. General Services Administration. Available at http://www.cfda.gov/public/writing.pdf/.

National Institutes of Health Office of Extramural Research. Award trends. Available at http://grants1.nih.gov/grants/award/awardstr.htm/.

National Institutes of Health Office of Extramural Research: available at http://www.grants.nih.gov/funding/funding_program.htm/.

Texas Researchers Administrators Group: available at http://tram.east.asu.edu/fund/foundation.html/.

Selected organizations

Agency for Healthcare Quality and Research (AHRQ)
John M. Eisenberg Building
540 Gaither Road
Rockville, MD 20850
http://www.ahrq.gov/

National Institutes of Health (NIH)
9000 Rockville Pike
Bethesda, MD 20892
http://www.nih.gov/

National Science Foundation
4201 Wilson Boulevard
Arlington, Vt 22230
http://www.nsf/gov/

WRITING FOR PUBLICATION

You have developed your research idea, written a protocol, and had it approved by the IRB. Then you wrote a grant and had it funded, conducted your research, and analyzed the data. Now you are ready to write the report for publication. This final, important step is the payoff. Yet, I wonder how many research projects wither in desk drawers simply because the investigators do not complete the final step—writing for publication. (Maybe this would be a good research question.)

The Publication Imperative

We have all heard the old saying that in universities, one must "publish or perish." In medical academics, I believe it is more like "publish or languish." Because you are a clinician, you will not really perish, but your academic career will suffer as you fail to receive the rewards of more "successful" faculty: recognition, invitations to speak at national meetings, grant awards, administrative assistance, even a new computer or better office. There is no question that medical writing is valued, especially reports of clinical studies that are published in refereed scientific journals.

It pays to start early to build up the publication list on your curriculum vitae (CV). At the end of a long academic career, those considered to have been most successful will have a trail of publications, just as Halley's comet has picked up a trail of dust in its wake. I recommend that you begin early, starting with review articles, case reports, book reviews, letters to the editor—anything to get some experience in medical publication.

Despite the well-recognized publication imperative, most faculty members spend little or no time writing during their first 3 years on faculty.[7] This is sad, because the early years of an academic career is exactly when you may have the most penetrating insights that could lead to innovative research or a thoughtful expository paper.

Do you require extra hours during the workday to accomplish your medical writing? Can you convincingly argue for "protected time?" This question has been studied, comparing faculty who publish and those who don't.[8] Published faculty members have no more discretionary time on their schedules than those who fail to publish. The difference seems to lie in the level of commitment and personal time management. Those who publish seem to build momentum that carries them to more success with each article in the literature.

The temptation, of course, will be to add to the burden of pedantic drivel that fills so many pages of scientific publications. For this reason, I challenge you as a young faculty member to maintain high standards and to put pen to paper (actually, today we open our laptops) only when you believe strongly that you have something important to share. Let the dust in the wake of your career shine as a credit to your scholarship.

Finding Information

One of the important skills in medical writing is being able to find information when you need it. Searching skills are important in both patient care and in writing for publication. You need to be able to do a rapid and comprehensive literature search when planning a research study in order to discover the state of the art for your chosen topic. You have the same need when describing the problem and structuring the rationale for your grant proposal or when writing for publication. For these reasons, I will discuss here some basic information-finding strategies that all academic clinicians should master:

Search Engines

There are a number of major search engines on the Web. These are used for searches of all types and can be helpful for some scientific writing projects. Major search engines include Google, Yahoo!, Ask Jeeves, Dogpile, and others.[9] I will discuss two briefly:

- **Google** (www.google.com) is my go-to search engine and the home page on my browser. Readers of Search Engine

Watch have voted Google the "Most Outstanding Search Engine" four times.[9] It claims to search more than 8 billion Web pages in its index. If you are not familiar with Google and if you are a published author, type in your name and the topic of your paper and see what you get. Google does not display pop-up ads, and the site seems to get a little better each month. Also, for "scholarly" information, check out www.scholar.google.com/.

■ **Dogpile** (www.dogpile.com) is a meta-search engine whose Web site claims that it "makes searching more of the Web easier by returning the best results from these leading engines: Google, Yahoo!, Ask Jeeves, About, LookSmart, Overture, FindWhat." If my Google search doesn't give me what I need, I often try Dogpile.

Medical Web Sites

There are a number of these; some are free and some are not. I'll discuss three of them. The search described was performed in January 2005.

■ PubMed (http://www.pubmed.com) is my favorite medical Web site. This is a service of the National Library of Medicine that allows you to search up to 14 million references in the biomedical sciences, including those in MEDLINE and others. I searched PubMed for "hypnic headache AND therapy." (Hypnic headache is a recently elucidated headache that causes nocturnal cephalgia and occurs chiefly in older persons.) My results were a list of studies that were very relevant to the topic and, in most instances, offered the option of going directly to the abstracts.

■ Medscape (http://www.Medscape.com) is a free Web site that offers access to MEDLINE. It also can provide specialty specific data and a no-charge e-mail address. I searched Medscape/MEDLINE for the same topic "hypnic headache AND therapy." The first three papers listed covered hypnosis and acupuncture, and not hypnic headache.

■ MDConsult (http://www.Mdconsult.com) is a fee-based
service that relies on approximately 40 medical reference
books and more than 50 top medical journals. What sets
it apart is the access to the reference books, which
can be especially useful in patient care on a busy day.
Good features are the drug information list and printable
patient handouts. I searched MDConsult for "hypnic
headache AND therapy," and here I found a helpful list
of journal articles on treating hypnic headache.

Writing the Report of a Clinical Study

There are many models of medical writing. These include
the case study, the review article, editorial, letter to the
editor, book review, book chapter, authored reference
book and more.[10] Here I will limit the discussion to what
I consider the most challenging model of medical writing—
the report of a clinical study. This model is difficult for
newcomers for several reasons: First of all, it is a report
of research you have done, and that means that you have
performed a clinical study and have some analyzed
data before you. Second, there is a strict protocol for
how the report should be written, and any deviation invites
rejection of your paper. Third, and most daunting of all, is
the series of hurdles you will face in getting your paper published. Space in the top journals is precious and, in your
quest for publication, your paper will be reviewed by your
peers in a manner that helps assure the quality of published
articles but that can seem quite frustrating to aspiring
authors.

The time-honored model of writing a report of clinical
research is described as the IMRAD model, an acronym for
introduction, methods, results, and discussion, presented
with brief annotations in Table 6.7.

The four items in Table 6.7 are the skeleton of the clinical research report. The flesh on the bones is the expanded
IMRAD model. Keep in mind the four key components as
we explore the expanded IMRAD and more, beginning with
selection of the title for the report. The following descrip-

TABLE 6.7. The IMRAD model for a report of clinical research

Introduction: Tells about the question you hope to answer
Methods: Describes the subjects you studied, what you did to them, and how you handled the data
Results: Reports what you found
Discussion: Tells what you think it all means

tion of the expanded **IMRAD** model is adapted from my book on medical writing.[10]

Title

The title is the "label" for the paper. The title must tell, more or less, what was studied. Craft your title with care; it is the one part of the paper that most of your intended audience is likely to read, and on the basis of the title, they will make decisions as to whether to read the abstract and maybe even the rest of the paper.

An early question the writer must answer is this: Should I reveal my conclusion in the title? I think that to do so will require a verb. Whimster writes: "I believe that readers need a verb in the title, such as a newspaper headline usually has, and that to be meaningful it should convey the message, as in: 'Rickettsial endocarditis is not a rare complication of congenital heart disease in dental practice: a report of five cases.'"[11] The current trend seems not to use verbs and to keep the study outcome a secret from the reader who peruses only titles. Today I received my current issue of the *New England Journal of Medicine*, with five "original articles," or reports of original research. None had a simple verb in the title or told me the key finding. For example, the was a report titled "Maternal and Perinatal Outcomes Associated with a Trial of Labor after Prior Cesarean Delivery." In the abstract I learn that, "A trial of labor after prior cesarean delivery is associated with a greater perinatal risk than is elective repeated cesarean delivery without labor, although absolute risks are low." But the title gives scant clue to this conclusion. (Landon MB et al. N Engl J Med 2004; 351;2581–2589).

Consider using a colon in your title, which allows you to present the general topic, followed by your specific findings. On a technical basis, the instructions for authors may prescribe a word or character limit for the title. Also, I believe that titles should not contain acronyms or abbreviations, no matter how widespread the author and editor consider their use.

Authors

The chief issues in authorship of a research report are generally twofold: First: Who is an author? And second: In what order will the authors be listed?

Question one is clearly answered in the Uniform Requirements for Manuscripts Submitted to Biomedical Journals: "Authorship credit should be based only on 1) substantial contributions to conception and design, or acquisition of data, or analysis and interpretation of data; 2) drafting the article or revising it critically for important intellectual content; and 3) final approval of the version to be published. Conditions 1, 2, and 3 must all be met. Acquisition of funding, the collection of data, or general supervision of the research group, by themselves, do not justify authorship."[12]

No department chair or research director should insist on being named as an author unless there has been a significant contribution to the study and to writing the paper. Adding the name of a prestigious senior faculty member as the final entry on a long author list might help the paper's chances of acceptance, but including the well-known name implies that person's active participation in the project. Gratuitous addition of an author name is ethically inappropriate.

The order in which authors will be listed on the paper should be decided very early in the process, generally during one of the first meetings of the research group planning the study. Changes in the rank order can be made later if contributions of individuals to the project do not turn out to be what was originally planned.

The first author should be the one who has done most of the work. Generally, this is the person who led the research team and who created the early drafts of the paper. From then on, authors should be listed according to how much they contributed to the study and the paper. As one whose last name begins with a letter at the end of the alphabet, I have never considered alphabetical listings of names to be fair to the Taylors, Whiteheads, and Zells of the world.

A quirk of citation listing holds that when the paper is used as a reference in other studies, if your paper has seven or more authors, only the first three will be named and the rest will join the *et al.* army of obscure authors.

Abstract

Next comes the abstract, which is an author-generated synopsis of the paper. I believe that the final version of the abstract should be the last item written, as these few paragraphs are the most read and hence the most important of the article. You want to be sure that your most important data and conclusions appear here.

In general, the abstract should mirror the IMRAD structure of the paper. That is, the paper's introduction, methods, results, and discussion (conclusions) should each be presented in a sentence or two, and many good abstracts have exactly four short paragraphs. According to the Uniform Requirements, "The abstract should state the purposes of the study or investigation, basic procedures (selection of study subjects or laboratory animals; observational and analytic methods), main findings (giving specific data and their statistical significance if possible), and the principal conclusions. It should emphasize new and important aspects of the study or observations."[12]

The current trend is for journals to require structured abstracts. This means that information in the abstract will be presented according to specific headings that differ a little with each journal. Some journals prefer abstracts with full sentences; others encourage the use of phrases, such as from a report in the *British Medical Journal* (Cluett ER, Pickering RM, Getliffe K, Saunders NJS. Randomized controlled trial of labouring in water compared with standard augmentation for management of dystocia in first stage of labor. Br Med J 2004;238:314–319):

> **Objectives:** To evaluate the impact of labouring in water during the first stage of labour on rates of epidural analgesia and operative delivery in nulliparous women with dystocia.
> **Design:** Randomised controlled trial.
> **Setting:** University teaching hospital in southern England
> **Participants:** 99 nulliparous women with dystocia (cervical dilation rate less than 1 cm/hour in active labor) at low risk of complications.

And so Forth

Later in the abstract, under "Results and Conclusions," the style changes from phrases to complete sentences.

Check the journal's instructions to authors carefully to see if the abstract must follow a specific format and if there is a word limit.

On a technical basis, abstracts tell about work that has been done and should be written in the past tense. In the spirit of intellectual integrity, the abstract must never contain a conclusion that is not discussed in the body of the paper.

Key Words

Key words can be what keep your report from being lost in the information jungle. They are part of the retrievability process that can contribute to the number of times your paper will be cited. In the instructions to authors, many journals will request that you submit 3 to 10 key words or short phrases. These will "assist indexers in cross-indexing the article and may be published with the abstract."[12]

Introduction

Finally we arrive at the I in IMRAD. The introduction should tell about the problem you set out to solve. In general terms, the introduction should cover three areas:

■ Problem statement: What is the general nature of the problem that merits valuable journal space and the reader's attention?

■ Background and work to date: What are the most pertinent published studies that relate to the problem?

■ The research question: What is the specific, focused question that you set out to answer? Perhaps there are two or even three related questions.

The Problem

The introduction classically opens with a broadly stated and virtually unassailable generalization about the problem. In the Langdon and colleagues report of a trial of labor following prior C-section (see page 170), the authors begin to discuss the problem as follows: "The overall rate of cesarean deliveries in the United States has risen dramatically, from 5% in 1970 to a high of 26% in 2002." Later they discuss medicolegal pressures and more stringent criteria for a trial of labor after cesarean delivery, which have "led to a substantial decline in the rate of vaginal birth after cesarean section, to 12.7% in 2002."

Background

Tell the key work that has been done on the topic to date. In the words of Uniform Requirements, "Give only strictly pertinent references. . . ."[12]

Research Question

Describe clearly the question you are trying to answer. One focused question is better than many. The question may be stated as a query or perhaps as a hypothesis but often is phrased as a statement of intent: In the study of trial of labor after prior cesarean section, the authors describe: "We conducted a multicenter observational study involving women with a prior cesarean delivery to assess the risks of uterine rupture and neonatal and maternal morbidity associated with a trial of labor as compared with repeated elective cesarean delivery."

Technical Issues

When writing your introduction, use the present tense when describing the general nature of the problem and the background work. Then the research question, if presented as a statement, is usually in past tense, as in the example above.

The Uniform Requirements advise that you "do not include data or conclusions from the work being reported,"[12] but not all journals hold rigidly to this rule.

Methods

The methods section, sometimes called "Participants and Methods" or perhaps "Methods and Materials," should describe a logical experimental approach. Because this section will present a number of topics, subheadings are often used. In the methods section of the Langdon and colleagues labor/cesarean delivery article, the methods section had three subheadings: "Study Design," "Definitions" (such as uterine rupture), and "Statistical Analysis."

Fundamentally, this section needs to tell about the subjects, what you did to them, and what statistical methods you used. Methods should not include numerical data, which should be presented in the results section. After writing the first draft of the methods section, ask yourself if what you are presenting allows *reproducibility*. That is, could a trained investigator replicate your study, given the information you have provided?

Subjects

Describe the subjects studied, including age, sex, and other important characteristics that may be pertinent to the study. The Uniform Requirements recommends, when such descriptors are important, that authors "should avoid terms such as 'race,' which lacks precise biological meaning, and use alternative descriptors such as 'ethnicity' or 'ethnic group' instead."[12]

Tell also if any potential subjects were excluded and, if there is a meaningful reason, why they were excluded.

Methods

Here you tell what was actually done to the subjects. Be sure to identify all drugs by generic name; adding the trade name is optional but is useful for the practicing clinician. Be sure to include doses and routes of administration.

Statistics

Describe statistical methods used, "with enough detail to enable a knowledgeable reader with access to the original data to verify the reported results."[12] This means identifying specific tests used. In the study on labor/cesarean delivery, the method/statistical analysis section begins, "Continuous variables were compared with the use of the Wilcoxon rank-sum test, and categorical variables with the use of the chi-square test or Fisher's exact test. . . ." (The previous sentence is an example of why I advocate having a statistical expert on your research team.)

The Uniform Requirements recommend that authors "Put a general description of (statistical) methods in the Methods section. When data are summarized in the Results section, specify the statistical methods used to analyze them."[12]

Results

What did you discover? Describe your findings in a logical sequence and do so fully, yet succinctly. The informed reader should be able to replicate the statistical analysis. Provide all data that were analyzed on the way to your conclusions, and show the outcomes of the statistical analysis that you described in the methods section.

I have sometimes said, only partly in jest, that the ideal results section has a single sentence, "The results are presented in Table 1," followed by a single, carefully crafted table. In reality, presenting research results is never this simple, but the use of tables and figures can help organize numbers in ways that cannot be accomplished in words. Keep in mind that tables and figures are expensive for the journal to produce and are a leading source of error. On balance, however, most results sections benefit from one or more tables or figures.

Be sure to submit a legend for each table or figure, and do not present data both in a table and also in the text. Pick one.

Discussion

In order for your article to be accepted for publication, the discussion must answer the "So what?" question. Your article should do so by telling the relationships among facts discovered, relating them to prior studies (the ones you mentioned earlier in the introduction), and postulating what it may all mean—the conclusions. Discuss the results, but do not restate what has already been said in the results section.

The Holy Grail in all of this is *generalizability*, a neologism that is not in *Dorland's Medical Dictionary* but that all researchers recognize. Does what you have found apply only to your group of subjects, a weakness of the small sample or the single-institution study? Or can the results found be generalized to similar patients elsewhere, the obvious advantage of the large, multicenter trial such as the labor/cesarean delivery study?

Tell any weaknesses of the study design, or readers in letters to the editor will surely point these out later. The discussion section is also where you should describe any factors that may have biased collection of the data, such as unexpected events, attrition of subjects, or midstudy changes in methods, such as terminating one of the study groups.

In the last paragraph (where many readers will go right after reading the abstract), present a summary of your conclusions and their implications for clinical practice, the generalizability of your findings. Write this paragraph very carefully. It represents the outcome of months of work.

References

Your references tell where you have obtained information and indicate your knowledge of prior work in the area of your research. A focused list of citations is more valuable to your reader—and to you, as author—than a very long list of vaguely related papers.

When using a reference citation to support a statement, be sure that you are conveying the actual meaning of the author. I have seen too many references used to support statements when the paper cited says something entirely different. The following are some other thoughts about article references:

- If in doubt as to format, use the style in the Uniform Requirements[12] or in the *New England Journal of Medicine*. This assures that your citations contain all information needed for any journal I know.
- Uniform Requirements recommends that you avoid citing abstracts as references.[12]
- If in doubt in listing the name of a journal, write it out, because—for example—"Psych" could mean psychiatry or psychology.
- By custom, a journal with a single word title, such as *Nature* or *Science*, is written in full and is not abbreviated.
- A paper accepted for publication but not yet published can be cited as "in press." If the paper is published before your article citing it goes to press, the citation can be updated in proof.
- Because the site of electronic citations can change, the author citing a Web site should print out a copy of the online material, in case it is requested later.
- Never cite a source you have not read and copied for your files.

Acknowledgments

Some papers have a final section listing those who assisted with the work. This includes "all contributors who do not meet the criteria for authorship, such as a person who provided purely technical help, writing assistance, or a department chair who provided only general support."[12]

If financial or material support has not been disclosed elsewhere, it should be included here.

Be sure all that you thank are pleased to be acknowledged and that they actually agree with the substance of the paper. Being mentioned allows readers to infer that those thanked support the data and conclusions. For this reason, you should have written permission from all persons listed in the acknowledgments. Some journals have specific online forms for this purpose; others will accept a signed note on a letterhead.

Some Thoughts About Writing for Publication

Good Writing and Poor Research

Good writing cannot disguise a poor research design. Spend time and effort early in planning your research carefully, seeking advice from experts. You will have plenty of time later to write and rewrite your report.

Time to Write

Finding time to write is a major challenge for academic clinicians. If you ask any well-published clinician, you are likely to hear that his or her writing is done on nights and weekends. Not everyone agrees, however. Johnson advises "regular" brief writing sessions and, by regular, she means "at least four to five times per week, up to daily—the same schedule as for aerobic exercise!" She counsels against what she calls "binge writing."[13] As for me, however, with patients, students, residents, meetings, grants, and various interruptions, I have always found it very difficult to find much writing time during my busy day in the AMC.

Perhaps it will be helpful to look at the phases of writing. I can collect articles and other reference material at irregular times. Also, once a piece has been written, I can revise my work in short bursts of effort. But for the real writing—the creation of the first draft—I require a stretch of quiet, uninterrupted time. With experience, you will discover the writing time that works for you.

Writing as a Team Sport

Research should almost always be done as a team; it is an exercise in learning and in mutual support. Writing, notably composition, is done in the old-fashioned way—one person sitting before a computer screen. This means that the research team must decide who will do the hard work of writing the first draft of the report. In the best of all possible worlds, this person is the principal investigator on the grant and the leader of the research team. Such an alignment of the stars minimizes the risk of a battle over first authorship on the paper.

Writing the first draft should follow one or more discussions in which the team reached agreement on the data to be presented and what can be concluded from the data. I suggest that the tables be done first and approved by the group before writing text. Once the first draft is written, the team will engage in wordsmithing, working to create the best paper possible without "squeezing all the juice from the orange."

Getting Started

Sometimes is difficult to get started. When faced with a blank computer screen, you and I tend to engage in "avoidance behavior"—getting coffee, sharpening pencils, dusting nonexistent lint off the computer screen, looking out the window, or wandering through your Microsoft Word thesaurus. When you see this happening, you must act. Write something, even if it is not the first paragraph. Write a précis of what will be included in the paper. Or use the WIRMS question: Ask yourself, "What I Really Mean to Say is. . . ." Then write down your response.

Getting Finished

At some time you and your team must cease rewriting, declare the paper done, and submit it for publication. Young researchers often perseverate over a paper too long. Do not let the perfect become the enemy of the good. At some time you must let a journal editor and reviewers see your work, especially important if your data are going out of date while still on your desk.

On a realistic basis, you will almost certainly have at least one more chance to revise your paper. It is highly unlikely that a prestigious peer-reviewed journal will accept your paper "as is" without revisions. Realistically, your best hope is a "conditional acceptance" letter, suggesting that you make certain changes and then resubmit the article for another review. Although this response may sound discouraging, this is actually a very favorable outcome, which promises a high likelihood of acceptance of the revised paper.

Dealing with Rejection

If you submit many research reports to refereed journals, you will soon become familiar with the rejection letter. When your paper arrives in the journal office the editor scans it, and if he or she considers that it is possibly acceptable by the journal, it is sent to several reviewers for their comments. If the paper seems to reflect a jumbled research method, unfathomable prose, or a topic not relevant to the journal, you will receive it back by return mail with a comment reflecting that, "The paper does not meet our needs at this time."

Most quality papers will be reviewed, and for the typical peer-reviewed journal, a majority will be rejected. Despite the many journals published, space on the printed page is precious. Table 6.8 tells common causes of rejection of submitted research reports.

If your article is rejected—and many will be—resist the temptation to write an angry letter to the journal editors and reviewers. Instead, read the reviewers' comments carefully, and then put the paper aside for a few days. After you have allowed emotions to subside, use the helpful reviewer comments to make the needed revisions, and then send a clean copy of the paper to the next journal on your list.

With patience and perseverance, there is a journal home somewhere for the well designed, carefully conducted, clearly reported clinical study.

TABLE 6.8. Common reasons why research reports are rejected by journals

Topic considered inappropriate for the journal's audience
Literature review that ignores important published studies
Research method that does not answer the research question
Discussion and conclusion that are inconsistent with the data
Poor article construction and prose
Suspected author bias or other ethical concerns

TABLE 6.9. Information sources about medical writing for publication

Articles, books and Web sites
   Callaham M, Wears RL, Weber E. Journal prestige, publication bias, and other characteristics associated with citation of published studies in peer-reviewed journals. JAMA 2002;287:2847–2850.
   Day RA. How to write and publish a scientific paper, 5th ed. Westport CT: Oryx; 1998.
   International Committee of Medical Journal Editors. Uniform requirements for manuscripts submitted to biomedical journals. Updated 2001. Available at http://www.icmje.org/.
   Iverson C. American Medical Association Manual of Style, 9th ed. Baltimore: Williams & Wilkins, 1998.
   King LS. Why not say it clearly? Boston: Little, Brown, 1978.
   Taylor RB. The clinician's guide to medical writing. New York: Springer-Verlag, 2005.

Selected organizations
   American Medical Writers Association (AMWA)
   40 West Gude Drive, Suite 101
   Rockville, MD 20850-1192
   http://www.amwa.org/

   European Medical Writers Association
   http://www.emwa.org/

   National Association of Science Writers, Inc.
   http://www.nasw.org/

Where to Learn More About Medical Writing

There are a number of useful resources to help you learn more about writing for publication; see Table 6.9.

REFERENCES

1. Heinig SJ, Quon AS, Meyer RE, Korn D. The changing landscape of clinical research. Acad Med 1999;74:725–745.
2. Hoff JT. Research by academic surgeons. Am J Surg 2003; 185(1):13–15.
3. Bauer DG. The "how to" grants manual: successful grant seeking techniques for obtaining public and private grants, 5th ed. Westport CT: Praeger, 2003, p. 63.
4. Freeman R, Weinstein E, Marincola E, Rosenbaum J, Solomon E. Competition and careers in bioscience. Science 2001;294: 2293–2294.

5. Kotchen TA, Lindquist T, Ehrenfeld E. NIH peer review of grant applications for clinical research. JAMA 2004;291: 836–843.

6. Center loses grant by slimmest of margins. Oregonian. 2003; Dec. 3: p. D2.

7. Boice R. The new faculty member. San Francisco: Jossey-Bass, 1992.

8. Boice R, Ferdinand J. Why academicians don't write. J Higher Educ 1984;55(5):567–582.

9. Search Engine Watch. Available at http://www.searchenginewatch.com/.

10. Taylor RB. The clinician's guide to medical writing. New York: Springer-Verlag, 2005, pp. 198–209.

11. Whimster WF. Biomedical research: how to plan, publish and present it. New York: Springer-Verlag, 1997, p. 105.

12. International Committee of Medical Journal Editors. Uniform requirements for manuscripts submitted to biomedical journals. Available at http://www.icmje.org.

13. Johnson SR. Becoming a productive academic writer. Academic Physician & Scientist. 2004; Nov.–Dec.: pp. 2–3.

7
Administrative Skills

Success in academic medicine requires more than excellence in clinical care, teaching, and scholarship. You are now part of a large organization, and you should learn basic administrative skills. In this chapter, I will deal with three domains of administrative abilities: personal time management, meeting behavior and strategies, and leadership skills.

TIME-MANAGEMENT SKILLS

Do you ever wonder how one person seems to get so much more done than the rest of us and yet always seems energetic and even well rested? The answer is likely to be that the individual practices good personal time management. This apparent super-human has learned the importance of getting the right things done, in the right order, and at the right time. He or she does not give up sleep or all social activities but instead has learned how to work smarter. The following are some useful time-management strategies and some classic wasters of your valuable time.

Table 7.1 lists 10 strategies that can help you work smarter.

What to Do: Actions to Help You Work More Efficiently

The productive academic clinician begins with a prioritized list of what should be done today. There is likely to be the meta-schedule: I have hospital rounds at 7 a.m., see patients in the clinic at 9 a.m., check e-mails just before lunch, teach students in a seminar from 1 to 3 p.m., return telephone calls and e-mail messages, and then have some free time at my desk before a day's-end check of my hospital patients. The day's to-do list tells the tasks I hope to accomplish before evening. Items may include working on the outline for a

TABLE 7.1. Strategies for effective personal time management

What to do
 Do organize your work area for maximum efficiency.
 Do your most important work first.
 Do your most important work at your best time.
 Do delegate work that is best done by others.
 Do learn how to say "No."

What not to do
 Don't do work (e.g., completing a survey) just because it shows up on
  your desk.
 Don't handle a piece of paper or e-mail message more times than
  necessary.
 Don't save unimportant stuff in your files or on your computer.
 Don't sign up for a listserve unless it vital to your job.
 Don't waste time on things that don't really matter.

lecture, returning a call to an insurance company about a patient, getting some budget information for a grant proposal, and reviewing galley proofs of an article for publication. The well-organized academic clinician finishes the day's planned work on time and goes home feeling fulfilled. If you finish a little early, reward yourself by leaving a few minutes early rather than staying at your desk filling time.

Organizing Your Work Environment

Efficient time management begins with logistics. Your professional work area is a key to your productivity. It helps to have a well-lit, clutter-free work area. Have available everything you will need: up-to-date computer, printer, dictionary, reference books, writing materials, telephone, and all the file folders you will work on today.

Make the best possible use of your personal computer calendar. This schedule is likely to have your day's activities listed by hour, as well as to-do lists and an ongoing reminder column. Learn to use these tickler files to be sure that you don't neglect important items.

A good project management technique is the "Chronological File," a series of folders—either paper or on your computer—labeled by the months of the year. In my "Chron File" folders I put items that need to be done each month.

When the first of the month arrives, I take out that month's folder and start work on the tasks I find noted there.

Doing Your Most Important Work First

Prioritize your work. Begin by asking yourself, "What really needs to be done today and is so important that I would stay late to be sure it is accomplished?" Be judicious and fair to yourself in what you put on today's A-list. Then identify those things it would be good to accomplish if time permits but are not sufficiently important to justify staying late—the B-list. Lastly, think about what you might accomplish if there is extra time at the end of the day and or between meetings.

Doing Your Own Work First

Place your personal projects high on the list, ahead of the requests of others unless there is a powerful reason to do otherwise. We live in symbiotic relationships with our colleagues in regard to all three domains of medical academia—clinical care, teaching and scholarship. We discuss challenging cases, comment on one another's papers, review each other's grants, fill in surveys, and complete faculty evaluations on our colleagues. Although these all are important and should be accomplished within a reasonable time, the efficient academician gets his or her own work done first.

Doing Your Most Important Work at Your Best Time

In his book on Harry S. Truman, Axelrod quotes the former president, "Most people don't know when the best part of the day is; it's the early morning."[1] Every year, at a national meeting, I present a seminar on leadership. At one point in the presentation, I discuss time management, and I ask the audience to self-identify if each is a morning-person, evening-person, or neither. Very consistently, about two thirds of the persons in the room raise their hands as morning persons, about one third are evening persons, and only a very few are "just good all day." I know that I am a very definite morning person, and I use my mornings to do my most important work. At the time I am typing these words on my computer, it is 8:20 a.m., and I know that I have only about four more hours of my "best time" left before I should move to something less creative than writing first drafts of book chapters.

Delegating Work Best Done by Others

One of the skills of working in an organization is learning how to work efficiently with your support staff. The ubiquity of computers today tempts us to work independently of administrative colleagues and our support staff, a tendency that might contribute to inefficiency.

We clinicians learn in training how to work collaboratively with nurses, clerks, laboratory technicians, and other patient-care colleagues. In the academic setting, there are analogous administrative support persons who can be a big help in your teaching and scholarly projects, if only you will learn how to work with them. A good starting point is a series of one-to-one meetings with the department administrator, clerkship coordinator, residency coordinator, grants coordinator, network coordinator, and the administrative assistant assigned to help you. These persons are likely to be as good at their administrative jobs as you are at being a clinician. Ask them how you and they can interact best together. The answers may surprise you and are likely to make you a more efficient academician.

Learning to Use the "No" Word

An aversion to using the "No" word is a weakness of many clinicians, including academicians. The job just offers so many enticing opportunities, and it is hard to pass up even one. Unfortunately, overcommitment is rampant among academic clinicians and contributes to inefficient personal time management. It can also lead to dithering, depression, burnout, and sometimes even divorce.

When I was new to academic medicine and much younger than I am now, I was assigned an administrative assistant (AA) who was somewhat older than I, had abundant institutional workplace savvy, and was not impressed at all with my academic credentials. She soon identified my tendency to overcommit and recognized the threat to my well-being (and hers, as my AA). Once a week she would come into my office and say, "All right, Dr. Taylor. We're going to practice the drill again. Watch my lips. Say, 'No!'" I learned a lot from her.

What Not to Do

Much of what is on the don't-do list concerns "stuff" on your desk and on your computer. There is a wonderful way to handle much of the paper that crosses your desk; it is the *compost pile*. Put in the compost pile all the surveys, memos, notices, and other items that others think you really need to read. Let them ferment, and then at some later date, look at the oldest papers in the pile. Just as you find with your mail after returning from a long vacation, many of the "urgent" items have taken care of themselves or are no longer relevant.

In Table 7.1, the last entry concerns things that really don't matter. This brings us to the classic time-wasters listed in Table 7.2.

Being unable to find things is one of the biggest time-wasters of all. Take the time to organize your files—both your paper files and your computer files—so that you can locate what you need when you need it. Periodically weed out items that are out of date or no longer needed. When I place a new item in my paper files, I try to throw away an old item; this helps keep the volume under control and only very rarely do I later miss the discarded item. When I encounter a truly outdated file on my computer, I delete rather than close it.

Some academic clinicians no longer answer their telephones, allowing them to maintain their concentration on

TABLE 7.2. Personal time-wasters in academic medicine: Five leading offenders

Disorganization: cluttered desk and files
Telephone interruptions
Drop-in visitors
Perseveration
Purposeless meetings

the task at hand and permitting them to screen calls by later reviewing the voicemail messages left. I have not adopted this practice, but as a courtesy I do not answer the telephone if I am meeting with someone in my office.

It may seem rude to close your office door, but closing the door is often a good idea if you are working on a project—such as a rough draft of a paper or a grant proposal—that needs an extended period of concentration. In such an instance, you might put a sign on the door that reads, "Working on a grant. Interrupt only in emergency."

Casual drop-in visitors can consume much of your day, especially if your office is geographically located on a busy hallway. No one likes to be rude, but you have work that needs to be done before you go home tonight. If possible, consider placing your desk and chair so that your back is to the door. This discourages eye contact with casual passers-by who want to discuss last evening's TV reality show. If you want to chat, go to the coffee room; your office is a place for work and sometimes for meetings.

If you are afflicted by a chatterer who has wandered into your office, try one of these ploys: Stand up and remain standing until the chatterer has finished talking; eventually he or she will become tired of standing and move on. Or invite the person to come with your as you go to get a glass of water, a maneuver that gets the idler out of your office.

Don't perseverate over a task. Inappropriately persistent attention to an undertaking can burn up hours for little gain. Learn to do the best job you can in the time allotted. Then declare it done, and move on to the next activity. This applies to medical writing projects, grant proposals, clinical reports, and any document being prepared for dissemination. Remember that at some time on the way to the Gettysburg battlefield, Abraham Lincoln must have concluded, "This speech may not be long, but it says what I need to say. I think I will stop writing and declare it done."

I am ending my section on time-wasters with meetings that really don't serve much purpose. Do your best to avoid membership on task forces and committees that hold long meetings that achieve little. Be especially reluctant to join committees that meet at your "best time"—that's morning for most of us. Not all meetings are bad, of course, and some are vitally important to your patients' well-being, your department, or your career. For the others, you can improve your personal efficiency and the effectiveness of the meeting by learning good meeting skills.

MEETING SKILLS AND BEHAVIOR

In American corporations and in academic medical centers (AMCs), billions of dollars are wasted each year on unproductive meetings, with the costs buried in the institutional budgets. On the other hand, in the corporate setting and academic institutions, meetings are often the key events that determine the fate of projects and give activities needed momentum. Yes, meetings sometimes actually get work done. The academic clinician who declares, "I hate all meetings" risks failure in achieving important objectives.

Meetings are of two kinds. The first involves two or perhaps three people, and these get-togethers are usually focused on a task. This section chiefly discusses the second type, the group meeting.

Fundamentally, group meetings are held for one of three purposes: Information, debate and refer, and decision making. *Information meetings* usually involve large groups of diverse persons and are intended to be sure that all have heard important facts and directives. *Debate and refer meetings* allow constituents to influence decisions by discussing issues, with the recognition that final decisions will be made by a department chair or a small leadership group at a later time. *Decision-making meetings* are the most challenging to manage and allow the most opportunity for mischief. Clinical practice group meetings and faculty meetings often involve decisions. A meeting agenda may include items that represent all three elements—information, discussion only, and decisions. When this occurs, the agenda could clearly indicate the action to be taken. As a faculty member attending a meeting, you (and others at the meeting) must be sure that all understand the meeting's purpose.

Meeting Attendees and Logistics

Meeting logistics have to do with who is included, where the meeting is held, and who sits where.

Who Is Invited to the Meeting?

If you are attending a regularly scheduled meeting of a standing committee—for example, your department's quality assurance or residency curriculum committee—the invitee list is usually not in question; it consists of the committee members. If the meeting scheduled is an issue-oriented, ad hoc meeting, and if a decision is to be made at the meeting, who is invited is crucial. Even more important is who is not. One distinction between influence and power is this. Influence is having your views represented when a decision is made; power is being at the table for the decision. If you have a stake in a program and a decision is being made, you must be at the meeting.

The Location of the Meeting

The site of the meeting has great significance. First let me discuss invited meetings. Who can summon whom to meetings has considerable significance in the AMC. When I wish to meet with someone of equal or higher rank, I go to that person's office as a courtesy. If, for example, you are a clinical department chair, there are a very limited number of persons who can summon you to a one-to-one meeting in his or her office; in most instances, these are the president or provost of the university, the dean, and the hospital director. All others who wish to meet with a clinical department chair should offer to come to the chair's office. Junior faculty members do not have the power of a department chair but should nevertheless pay attention to where meetings occur, especially one-on-one meetings with another person.

Some of the same protocol holds with larger ad hoc meetings. It is always powerful to have an interdisciplinary meeting in your own departmental setting, giving you a "home-court advantage." If you are scheduling an inter-departmental meeting, going to a neutral site is respectful. Whatever you decide, where meetings are held matters.

Round Table or Square Table

I have been honored to serve as visiting professor at medical centers in several Asian countries, and these visits always involve at least one formal dinner. At these dinners, I soon learned that there is a rigid seating protocol based upon the "honored guest" tradition and the relative power of others at the table. It is the same with organizational meetings.

The power seats vary with the shape of the table and configuration of the room. In general, the seat facing the door is considered powerful. If a long, banquet-style table, the power seat will be in the middle of the table, not at the very end. If the table is a large square, as is often the case in hotel meeting rooms, the power seat will be in front of the white board or flip chart. Sitting with your back to the window is better than sitting with your back to the door. The weakest seats are in the corners of an open square or at the far corners of a long banquet table when the leader is seated in the middle.

Participating in a Meeting

Meeting Strategies

Table 7.3 tells strategies for effective meeting participation.

Effective participation in a meeting begins with preparation. Read the agenda in advance. Perhaps do some home-

TABLE 7.3. Strategies for effective meeting participation

What to do
    Do prepare for the meeting.
    Do arrive on time.
    Do find a "power seat" if one is available.
    Do know what you want from the meeting.
    Do feel free to challenge ideas.

What not to do
    Don't be the first to speak on an issue, unless you have a very good
        reason to speak first.
    Don't dominate the discussion.
    Don't criticize a proposal without a good idea to suggest.
    Don't ever attack anyone personally.
    Don't lose control of your emotions during a meeting.

work on the issue to be discussed. If you think it might be appropriate, bring handouts on important material; be sure you have enough handouts for everyone in the room. Then arrive early so that you don't have to take the last seat left in the room.

Never go into a decision-making meeting without knowing exactly what you want from the meeting. This may include planning a "fall-back position" and a strategy to divert discussion (such as to a small group to study the problem) if things are not going well.

Seasoned academicians are rarely the first to comment on a motion or new idea put before the group. They leave that risky action to the young and inexperienced. Veterans also don't talk too much in meetings, perhaps having learned, as President Lyndon Johnson once said, "When you are talking, you aren't learning anything."

Resist the urge to criticize ideas without a realistic alternative. If you think that a plan to change an administrative assistant's duties or a scheme to revise the faculty evaluation system is a bad idea, you really should have something better to propose.

Whatever happens, remember that you are a professional. Resist any urge to react to what happens in the meeting with an emotional outburst. Stay under control, and plan your long-term strategy, a much better alternative than undermining your credibility with what will surely be perceived as hysterics.

Comments and Questions for Meeting Participants

In academics we tend to meet with the same persons over and over, and we come to recognize their meeting strengths and weaknesses. We tend to listen carefully to those with good meeting skills and to favor what they recommend. For these reasons, you should learn how to be an effective meeting participant, which often means making the right facilitative comment at the right time. Some helpful meeting comments and questions are listed in Table 7.4.

TABLE 7.4. Effective meeting participation: Some helpful comments and questions

Is there possibly a new way to think about this issue?
Who outside this room should be included in the discussion?
Is what we are proposing consistent with our mission?
Can we accomplish our objectives with the available budget?
Is there a way to get outside funding for this project?
Should we appoint a small group to study the issue in depth and report back next meeting?
Let us not forget about our students (or residents, or patients). Have we considered what is best for them?
Have we considered the long-term implications?
I wonder if. . . .
How will we evaluate the outcome and measure success?

Chairing a Meeting

You may be charged with chairing a meeting because it is your turn in rotation, or because you head a committee or task force. In either case, you need to schedule the meeting, plan the agenda, and then conduct the meeting in a way that achieves the desired outcomes and is fair to all.

Table 7.5 summarizes ten strategies for chairing a meeting.

Scheduling a Meeting

Regular meetings occur at predictable times that should have already been reconciled with everyone's schedules.

TABLE 7.5. Strategies for effectively chairing a meeting

What to do
Do plan the agenda carefully.
Do arrive early for the meeting.
Do be sure that each agenda item gets its fair share of time.
Do try to see that everyone present gets a chance to speak.
Do encourage open discussion of the issues.

What not to do
Don't let the first agenda item use up all the agenda time.
Don't let one person dominate the discussion.
Don't allow the discussion to stray too far off the agenda.
Don't permit personal attacks.
Don't forget to conclude the meeting on time.

Special meetings need careful negotiation to find times when all stakeholders can attend. In the AMC, this is often early morning, lunchtime, or at 5 p.m.

Planning a Meeting Agenda

The agenda should guide what happens at the meeting, and the chair should try to follow the planned agenda as closely as possible. Sticking to the agenda helps assure that everyone's expectations are met. Those who will participate in the meeting should be surveyed before the meeting, asking for items to be discussed. Then the chair uses these to construct the agenda.

As suggestions are melded into an agenda, you must be careful to allot time appropriately. Remember that any discussion can last much longer than anticipated. For this reason, you should plan the sequence of items with care. If possible, plan to move from easier to more difficult items during the meeting and allot a designated time for each discussion. It is best to err on the side of covering too few items than too many.

The agenda should be prepared several days before the meeting and then sent to all who will attend. At that point, someone may want to amend the agenda, but as chair, you might politely inform that person that everyone had a chance for input earlier.

Conducting the Meeting

The meeting should begin exactly at the scheduled hour to respect those who came on time. Confirm with the participants the time allocations for various agenda topics, because you intend to adhere to them. Preview the objectives for the meeting: For example, "When we finish in one hour, we should have a yes or no decision on approving Bill's grant proposal and we should have had a good discussion of the new weekend call rotation before referring to Mary to draw up the actual schedule."

The chair must keep the discussion on the topic. Do not hesitate to call, "Time out. We are getting off the topic. Who has a comment on the topic we are discussing?"

Effective chairing also means being sure that everyone gets his or her fair share of "air time." Those who talk too much may be balanced by asking the quiet ones for their comments. Any hint of a personal attack can be controlled by requesting a return to addressing the issue, not the individual.

Some meeting chairs like to use strict parliamentary procedure, but in the AMC, most do not. Sometimes chairs will summarize comments on a flip chart, which can help structure the discussion. Another maneuver of some chairs is to appoint a timekeeper to monitor the time allocations of the agenda items. A chair may choose to comment on some or all contributions, but this always seems somewhat controlling to me. Whatever techniques are used, the meeting chair should encourage and model problem-solving behavior, focusing on facts and seeking balance among conflicting opinions.

At the end, the chair should summarize what has been decided at the meeting and then conclude on time. A written record of the meeting—the minutes—should follow within a few days. The chair should carefully review and edit the minutes before they are distributed. Preparing minutes of the meeting is occasionally more than a clerical chore; in contentious situations, I have seen instances in which the person who wrote the meeting's minutes controlled the long-term outcome of the meeting.

Best Meeting Behavior

The following are some observations about meetings that I did not cover above.

Supportive Phrasing Even When You Disagree

Sometimes you just must disagree. There has been a budget cut and your colleague wishes to solve the problem by dismissing a key administrative assistant. As a skillful meeting participant you might say, "Yes, I can see the reasoning behind your proposal. But let's consider another way to cover the deficit, such as each of us scheduling one additional patient visit in the clinic each day." You have validated the person as a reasonable thinker while offering an alternative suggestion.

Destructive Comments

Negative comments can cause a pall to descend on the meeting. The speaker assumes an aggressor role and the recipient becomes a victim. Progress in the meeting becomes stalled until equilibrium is restored. Table 7.6 lists some classic destructive comments.

Dealing with the Bully

We can all recognize bullying behavior in a meeting. The bully interrupts, speaks rudely to one person or to everyone, and engages in dominating body language. Sometimes you need to confront the bully. I saw this done effectively some years ago in a meeting of clinical department chairs. The bully was a senior chief of a surgical service who had already held court in the meeting too long. Then came the turn to speak of a newly arrived, somewhat younger chair of another department. In the middle of the new chair's second sentence, the bully interrupted and began speaking loudly. I watched as the new, young chair sat up straight, lowered his voice a little, looked at the bully and said, "Dr. Jones, I sat and listened respectfully while you talked. Now it is my turn, and I hope that you will sit and listen until I finish." The mouths of everyone in the room dropped. No one had ever spoken to the senior surgeon this way. But he sat quietly, and he did not interrupt again.

Distracting Behavior

When you are in a meeting, everyone is aware of what everyone else is doing. Do not shuffle papers, talk to your neigh-

TABLE 7.6. Destructive comments heard at meetings

I don't like this proposal at all and I don't know why we're even discussing it.
We tried this in the past and it didn't work.
Whose dumb, crazy, idiotic idea was this?
This will never succeed.
I don't care about the rest of you; I will never support this decision.

---

bor in a side conversation, or play with your wireless mail device.

Translating Decisions into Action

Meeting chairs or management leaders can subvert the outcomes of meetings by exerting what Mankins calls a "pocket veto."[2] When this happens, there is debate in the meeting, decisions are reached, minutes are written and circulated, and then nothing occurs. Eventually everyone goes on to new topics and forgets that there ever was consensus reached on an issue. One of the duties of an effective chair is to help prevent the pocket veto of important decisions made in meetings.

Burying Bad Decisions

Sometimes groups of very smart professionals make bad decisions—approving proposals that, if implemented, would be disastrous. When you become aware that a Bad Decision has been made, there is one last maneuver that can avoid group self-destructive behavior. This tactic is the called the "Death by Legal Review" gambit. Dilbert describes this eloquently: "From time to time it will be necessary to kill a project without being identified as the assassin. That's why [AMCs] have legal departments."[3] No project is so benevolent, logical, and risk-free that your AMC lawyer can't kill it. Thus, when you recognize a potentially disastrous group decision, urge that the AMC legal department review the project prior to implementation.

What Meetings Really Represent

As I close the discussion of meetings, I want to share Lewis Thomas' notion of meetings as theater. ". . . when committees gather, each member is necessarily an actor, uncontrollably acting out the part of himself, reading the lines that identify him, asserting his identity. This takes quite a lot of time and energy, and while it is going on, there is little chance of anything else getting done."[4] Well, maybe there is hope. Perhaps something good will happen if there is good leadership.

LEADERSHIP SKILLS

Leadership and management skills are needed when you assume administrative responsibility for a meeting, teaching program, hospital service, research team, clinical section, or academic department. Souba writes, "Leadership is a uniquely human activity—studying it and how it works is core to the learning organization."[5] The study of leadership today has evolved from just looking at the characteristics of "the top dog" to a systems view that embraces the optimal deployment of individual and organizational capital, the dynamics of negotiation and resource exchange, and the process of positioning the institution for future growth.

About Leadership Today

Leadership is defined by what is done. Leaders influence behavior of persons and organizations. I believe that, in general, effective leaders perform three linked functions: First of all, they can *envision* how the world can be better. Then they *communicate* that vision to those who will be followers. Finally, leaders *energize* the followers to join in the quest to make the vision a reality. Leadership is a job that requires commitment and vigor. It is also sometimes a lonely job, one reason being that, metaphorically, the prototypical leader lives in a different time warp than other people. He or she can see tomorrow in ways that others cannot.

Although the words are often, and incorrectly, used interchangeably, leadership and management are different. Leadership is about vision, possibilities, theory, and change. Management skills are about practicality, facts, implementation, and rules. Managers promulgate rules and assemble three-ring binders with directives and regulations; leaders see regulations as obstacles to be overcome on the way to achieving a vision. I think of leaders building castles in the sky and managers charging rent on the castles. Successful organizations require both leaders and managers, ideally with the leader as the chief executive officer (and perhaps the founder) and the manager as the chief operating officer who makes things happen day by day.

We still debate whether the ability to lead is imprinted at birth or is teachable and learnable. Certainly, some classic leaders—Ghengis Khan, Jesus of Nazareth, Martin Luther King, and Gandhi—had gifts that you or I do not. On the other hand, according to Dwight Eisenhower, "The one quality that can develop by studious reflection and practice is the leadership of men."[6] If there is hope for most of us to rise to leadership roles in academic medicine, we must believe that leadership can be a learned skill.[7]

It would be tempting to continue writing about leadership theory and practice, but there are many excellent books on the topic. Table 7.7 provides a short annotated bibliography

TABLE 7.7. Selected books about leadership

Bennis W, Nanus B. Leaders: the strategies for taking charge. New York: Harper & Row, 1986.

    Thoughtful organization, crisp style, and clear thinking characterize this book. Much of their leadership theory concerns power and empowerment. A one-sentence synopsis of the book is found on page 86: "... nothing serves an organization better — especially during times of agonizing doubts and uncertainties — than leadership that knows what it wants, communicates those intentions, positions itself correctly, and empowers its work force." Bennis and Nanus developed the concept of "leading others, managing yourself."

Collins JC, Porras JI. Built to last: successful habits of visionary companies. New York: Harper Collins, 1997.

    The authors of this book (according to the Preface) "set out to discover the timeless management principles that have consistently distinguished outstanding companies." Examples include Boeing, Merck, and Walt Disney, which the authors call "visionary companies." Many of the concepts described could apply to leading academic practice groups and professional organizations.

Giuliani RW. Leadership. New York: Hyperion, 2002.

    Familiar to all Americans for his leadership during the September 11, 2001, crisis, Rudolph Giuliani tells his principles for leadership, using personal stories as examples.

Hickman CR. Mind of a manager; soul of a leader. New York: John Wiley & Sons, 1990.

    This book is for those seeking an in-depth differentiation between management and leadership.

TABLE 7.7. *Continued.*

Koch R. The 80/20 Individual. New York: Doubleday, 2003.
  Using Pareto's 80/20 principle, Koch discussed effective time management, telling ways to actually accomplish more by doing less.
Kouzes JM, Posner BZ. The leadership challenge: how to get extraordinary things done in organizations. San Francisco: Jossey-Bass, 1995.
  In preparation for this book, the authors collected questionnaires completed by more than 550 managers. Each was asked to describe his or her personal best leadership experience and answer a number of other open-ended questions. The book builds on these data, supplemented by interviews, by describing five practices of exemplary leadership (challenging the process, inspiring a shared vision, enabling others to act, modeling the way, and encouraging the heart) and telling how these practices can be transformed into action.
Northouse PG. Leadership: theory and practice, 2nd ed. Thousand Oaks, CA: Sage Publications, 2001.
  This book is intended to bridge the gap between popular approaches to leadership and more abstract theories. The author addresses topics such as situational leadership, contingency theory, path-goal theory, transformational leadership, and team leadership. Cases are used to illustrate concepts. The book presents a solid overview and is written in a style that would be useful as a course text.
Perkins DNT. Leading at the edge: leadership lessons from the extraordinary saga of Shackleton's Antarctic expedition. New York: American Management Association, 2000.
  In 1914, explorer Ernest Shackleton and his men were stranded on the Antarctic floes when their ship was crushed by an expanding ice pack. The group was rescued 2 years after their departure. This book seeks to identify leadership principles that helped Shackleton lead his team to safety.

of books on leadership; some are classic and general and others are current and specialized. For the remainder of this section, I will focus on what's special about leadership in academic medicine.

Leadership in the Academic Medical Center

What is special about leadership in the AMC that might be a little different than leadership in your town council, a sports team, a church group, the state legislature, or even General Motors? Allowing that there are many commonalities with nonacademic organizations, I believe that some distinctive characteristics are found in medical academics in the following areas: how we think about leadership, the academic leader's constituency, connectivity in academic leadership, the types of power and influence academic leaders hold, leadership styles that work, the role of negotiation in academic leadership, and the process of planning for tomorrow.

How We Think About Leadership

Academic medical centers produce a product—new knowledge (see Chapter 3). The also provide service, notably teaching and patient care. The integration of generating knowledge and providing service in diverse health-related fields demands high-level, innovative, and collaborative leadership.

Leaders shape the AMC's destiny. A president, provost, or dean recruits the best possible department chairs to the institution. These chairs, in turn, recruit what they hope will be hard working and innovative faculty, and there is a not-so-subtle competition to have each clinical department outshine the others just a little. Witness the classic sibling rivalry between the surgeons and the internists, the "technicians" versus the "cognitive doctors." Within each department, there are those who are primarily clinicians and there are the researchers. Leaders who can make these eagles fly in formation are a valued organizational resource.

Based on research, McCall identifies three traits of successful leaders in professional organizations[8]:

- **Maintaining technical competence.** If I am a skilled corporate leader or manager, I might move from a company manufacturing machine tools to one moving sports equipment from city to city, and later to another selling auto parts. I don't need to know how to actually make any of the products; I need to know how to lead (or manage), generic organizational skills that are transferable among many industries. Academic medicine is different in that a chairman of surgery is expected to perform operations and a chairwoman of obstetrics and gynecology will probably deliver babies, all while leading complex departments with multimillion-dollar budgets. The continuing technical competence gives these leaders credibility and also lets them use current, real-world experience in solving problems and relating to colleagues in the community.

■ **Promoting group decision-making**. One of my early mentors in academic administration characterized the AMC leadership role as *shaping consensus*. Clinicians and other academic professionals are generally bright and independent thinkers. They bristle at directives and instead want keenly to understand the reasons for decisions. They value participative decision-making, and in this setting, the leader is challenged to orchestrate the best decision for the organization with the "buy-in" of members of the group.

■ **Providing a work challenge**. Few in academic medicine at any level would be satisfied doing highly repetitive, mind-numbing assembly-line work no matter what the salary. Academic clinicians are highly educated and often fiercely motivated, and they value an opportunity to create and contribute. The best leaders provide this challenge, which to many is more valuable than high salary or the other rewards of academic medicine that I discussed in Chapter 3.

Constituency Issues in Academic Leadership

If I led a company making automobile tires, I would be in charge of managers and workers. We would be committed to one mission—make the best tire possible. Our objective is to make a profit for the stockholders. The focus is very clear. I would have four main constituencies: my shareholders, the management team, the workers who actually make the tires, and the customers who drive on them.

In academic medicine, just to review, we provide clinical care, teach learners of various types, and create new knowledge. Hence the academic leader's constituents are patients and their families; students, residents, and community physicians (the latter desiring continuing medical education); and a variety of faculty members and staff that will probably include physicians, researchers, educators, nurses, administrative employees, and more. These are broadly diverse constituencies, with widely varied education and training, career objectives, work ethics, values, and perceptions of where resources should be committed. The task of the academic leader is to unite these constituencies to achieve well-chosen objectives.

The Connectivity of Academic Leadership

In Chapter 3, I showed how the organizational structure could seem unfathomable and unworkable and so arcane it would cause Einstein to throw up his hands in dismay (see Figure 3.1). Yet this very organizational dysfunction serves a useful purpose in that it fosters connectivity.

A generation ago, academic medical centers consisted of departmental fiefdoms, ruled by what some considered "warlord chairmen." Today, thanks in part to new technology and also to some disease (not specialty) oriented grant programs, the departmental barriers are breaking down a little, and we are seeing multidisciplinary centers on women's health, cancer, bone and joint disease, heart disease, digestive diseases, and more. No single specialty controls these centers, and their success depends on the leadership abilities of various specialists to maintain the sometimes-fragile interdepartmental partnerships.

Power and Influence in Academic Leadership

Philosopher Bertrand Russell once remarked that, "The fundamental concept in social science is power, in the same sense in which energy is the fundamental concept in physics."[9] The concept of power can be viewed in various ways. One is the notion of potential and actual force. The electrical plug in the wall behind you holds electrical power, which you may or may not choose to use to turn on a light. If you use the power, you create a force that is consuming energy, a potentially exhaustible resource. In the same sense, leadership power can be implemented—or can be retained as a potential force. Power used is power lost, in the sense that the academic leader who uses power repeatedly, or even capriciously, may soon find that the power is gone.

In another sense, leadership represents formal authority to direct the actions of others. In April 1956, at Parris Island, South Carolina, a Marine drill instructor ordered the recruits of Platoon 71 to march into water over their heads. They did so, even though some of them could not swim and six of them subsequently drowned.[10] No group of academic clinicians would consider obeying any apparently pointless command, especially one that might prove dangerous. They would demand to know the logic behind the order and the intended objectives. There is no unquestioning obedience in the AMC. In fact, the faculty members would probably debate the merits of the marching order until the drill instructor gave up in frustration.

Power in academic medicine requires the positive traits described above, especially technical competence. It demands skill in developing group consensus and in motivating productivity. But, and probably most of all, power in academic leadership requires trust. Trust, the glue that holds organizations together, is what allows academic faculty to accept decisions that might reduce their salaries, increase their work hours, or even doom their favorite projects. Such decisions can be accepted, albeit reluctantly, if they trust the leader's motives and if they have confidence in the decision-making process.

Leadership Styles in Academic Medicine

In business, we often see autocratic styles. Lee Iaoccca typified this style, as does Donald Trump. In politics we have seen dictators such as Saddam Hussein and Fidel Castro, and also parental leaders such as Ronald Reagan. We have also marveled at the charismatic leaders such as Martin Luther King and John F. Kennedy. In academic medicine, none of these styles works very well for long. In a setting where success depends, more than anything, on convincing highly intelligent, yet independent, people to work together, what works is a facilitative leadership style. Facilitative leaders are those who live by the motto, "You can change the world if only you don't care who gets credit." This type of leader can bring key persons to the table to struggle to consensus. The facilitative leader seeks organizational excellence by helping each constituent reach his or her full potential. If you think of the most successful academic leaders you know, and those who have enjoyed the longest tenure, you will probably bring to mind a list of facilitative leaders.

Negotiation in Academic Medicine

Leadership and management in academic medicine is often concerned with the deployment of shared scarce resources. These include department budgets, office space, curriculum time, administrative support, research assistance, and travel opportunities. Getting your department's or program's fair share of resources or adjudicating conflict about access to these resources demands that academic leaders hone their negotiation skills.

Getting your fair share of resources for you and your constituents may involve what I call *anticipatory negotiation*. This means making a concession even before there is a negotiation—doing a favor with no demand for anything in return. It means teaching in a course sponsored by another department. It means covering a hospital service for another team so that they can attend a holiday party. It sometimes means letting another take credit for something you have done. It is building a stack of "credibility chips."

Cohen describes this as the reciprocity norm—performing an act that the other will feel an urge to match. He goes on to describe the observations of the French sociologist Alexis de Tocqueville that Americans adhere to a doctrine of enlightened self-interest. "When he asked one of our ancestors why he risked his life running into a burning house to save the children of a stranger, he got this reply: 'Well, by doing it, I expect someone would do the same for me someday.'"[11]

But anticipatory negotiation is often not enough, and it merely sets the stage for the give-and-take that a leader needs when deciding who gets what, and when, and under what circumstances. To be an effective negotiator in your role as an academic leader, you will need to cultivate the following traits:

■ **Confidence.** You must come to the table believing that your position is fair to all, that you can deliver what you promise, and that your team supports you.

■ **Preparation.** Never come to a bargaining table without knowing what you want, what you are willing to give up, and when you might be prepared to walk away from the proposal.

■ **Organization.** You must be able to structure choices in a way that ideas are readily understood and that options are clearly stated.

■ **Optimism.** Begin with the belief that agreement can be reached amicably.

■ **Collaboration.** Assume that what brings you to the bargaining table is a shared problem.

■ **Rationality.** Be able to care about the issue but not to the degree that you make harmful concessions just to close a deal.

In all critical negotiation, leaders should come to the table knowing their BATNA—the "Best Alternative to a Negotiated Agreement."[12] The BATNA can change over time, as you learn more facts in the negotiation, especially about how much emotion the other side brings to the discussion and how a decision will be made. For example, imagine that you are director of a university-affiliated outpatient clinic. Because of budget cuts, your chair must reduce your operating expenses by $250,000, beginning 2 months from now. A budget reduction of this magnitude could only mean that several persons would lose their jobs. In your opinion, this cut is unfair, and reductions should instead be made in other areas of the department budget. You go to meet with the department chair on behalf of your clinic's physicians and staff. Your goal is to have the proposed cut rescinded. "Not possible." Can the cut be reduced? "No." Can you have more time to try to increase income? "No." You are encountering a stone wall in your attempts to eliminate or reduce the budget cut. What should you do next? Should you make plans to fire some physicians and staff members? Should you threaten to quit your job? With a failed negotiation, what you do now is your BATNA.

Planning for Tomorrow in the AMC

Benjamin Franklin said that, "If you fail to plan, you are planning to fail." I believe that planning for tomorrow's AMC leadership involved both a mega-strategy and a micro-strategy. The mega-strategy involves systems thinking. Whatever your leadership role in the AMC, think of yourself as serving the mission of the institution. If what you are doing does not serve this mission, ask yourself if perhaps you should redirect your efforts. For example, are you serving the institution's best interest if you lead a public protest against a painful economic decision that the university was forced to make, such as closing a neighborhood clinic? Is there a better way to exert your influence within the system that will not undercut your leaders?

An interesting feature of systems leadership in the university is how the effective leaders at all levels come to work outside of their departments and for the common good. In the book *Good to Great*, Collins describes what makes companies into superstars. He describes levels of leadership, with the top leaders distinguished by their focus not on themselves but on the organization.[13] When I first became a clinical department chairman, I spent the first few years working hard to recruit outstanding faculty and making our department successful; then I found that increasingly my work took me outside the department to work for the greater good of the institution—the organizational system orientation.

At the other end of the spectrum, we work to assure the institution's future by nurturing tomorrow's leaders. This calls for recruiting young faculty with leadership potential, giving them jobs that promote their abilities, and affording them increasing authority as they develop task-related maturity. We need to act as administrative mentors, as well as research and career mentors. Young faculty in new leadership roles must be protected from administrative overload and burnout and should be rewarded for taking risks and for every success.

Today's young physicians recognize the need for leadership training. In a survey of surgery residents regarding 18 leadership skills, more than half of the respondents rated themselves as not competent or only minimally competent in 10 of the 18 areas listed. Yet, 92% rated all 18 leadership skills as somewhat or very important for career development.[14] There are a number of leadership training programs available to academic faculty, including the Hedwig van Ameringen Executive Leadership in Academic Medicine (ELAM) Program for Women,[15] Academic Physicians and Leaders (APALs) training[16] and various seminars available through the Association of American Medical Colleges (AAMC).[17]

In their book *In Search of Physician Leadership*, LeTourneau and Curry write, "Once the decision-making captains, both clinically and administratively, of the healthcare ship, physicians have seen their authority and influence slip over the past decades. It should be no surprise, then, that physicians are showing an increasing interest in regaining some of the control they have lost, especially to non-physicians."[18] Perhaps with the new generation of

TABLE 7.8. Information sources about academic administrative skills

Articles and books

    Allen D. Getting things done: the art of stress-free productivity. New York: Penguin, 2003.

    Emergency medicine: an academic career guide. Lansing, MI: The Society for Academic Emergency Medicine, 2000.

    McCabe LRB, McCabe ER. How to succeed in academics. New York: Academic Press, 2000.

    LeTourneau B, Curry W. In search of physician leadership. Chicago: Health Administration Press, 1998.

    McKenna MK, Pugno PA. Physicians as leaders: who, how, and why now? Abingdon UK: Radcliffe Publishing, 2005.

Web sites

    Centers of Leadership in Academic Medicine: available at http://www.4woman.gov/owh/col/.

    Time Management for the Academic Emergency Physician: available at http:www.emedicine.com/emerg/topic673.htm/.

Selected organizations

    American College of Physician Executives: available at http://www.acpe.org/index.htm/.

    Association of Academic Medical Colleges, Group on Faculty Practice: available at http://www.aamc.org/members/gfp/.

leadership-savvy clinician faculty, we will see a shift back toward having AMC decisions about clinical care, teaching, and scholarship guided by clinicians.

WHERE TO LEARN MORE ABOUT ADMINISTRATIVE SKILLS

Table 7.8 presents selected resources to help you learn more about academic administrative skills.

REFERENCES

1. Axelrod A. When the buck stops with you: Harry S. Truman on leadership. New York: Penguin Books, 2004, p. 279.
2. Mankins MC. Stop wasting valuable time. Harvard Business Review 2004; September: pp. 58–65.
3. Adams S. The Dilbert principle. New York: Harper Collins, 1996, p. 88.
4. Thomas L. The Medusa and the snail. New York: Viking Penguin Books, 1974.
5. Souba WW. New ways of understanding and accomplishing leadership in academic medicine. J Surg Res 2004;117: 177–186.
6. Ambrose SE. Eisenhower, Volume 1. New York: Simon & Schuster, 1983.
7. Taylor RB. Leadership as a learned skill. Family Pract Mgt 2003;10(9):43–46.
8. McCall MW. Leadership and the professional. Greensboro NC: Center for Creative Leadership, 1981.
9. Bertrand Russell quotation: Available at http://www.borntomotivae.com/BertrandRussell/html/.
10. Platoon #71, Parris Island, 1956. Available at http://www.au.af.mil/au/awc/awcgate/usmchrist/parris.txt/.
11. Cohen H. Negotiate this. New York: Warner Business Books, 2003, p. 130.
12. Why is BATNA important? Available at http://www.negotiationskills.com/qaprocess12.html/.
13. Collins JC. Good to great. New York: HarperBusiness, 2001.
14. Itani KM, Liscum K, Brunicardi FC. Physician leadership is a new mandate in surgical training. Am J Surg 2004;187: 328–331.
15. The Hedwig van Ameringen Executive Leadership in Academic Medicine (ELAM) Program for Women. Available at http://www.drexel.edu/elam/home.html/.

16. Fairchild DG, Benjamin EM, Gifford DR, Huot SJ. Physician leadership: enhancing the career development of academic physician administrators and leaders. Acad Med 2004; 79(3):214–218.

17. Association of American Medical Colleges. Seminars. Available at http://www.aamc/org/meetings/.

18. LeTourneau B, Curry W. In search of physician leadership. Chicago: Health Administration Press, 1998.

8
Academic Medicine Success Skills

The human beings in an academic medical center (AMC) exist in a complex social order that, like any such multifaceted organization, is composed of a small group at the top and a much larger group that report to them while they carry out their daily tasks. The same structure is mirrored in each academic clinical department. The small group at the top of the AMC hierarchy or in a department is there by a process of social Darwinism and not by chance. Some factors that help clinicians rise in the academic hierarchy are specialty choice: Specialists in internal medicine hold many deanships. Some have extra credentials, such as a master of business administration (MBA) degree as well as an MD degree. Others have had rapid career advancement owing to time spent at the National Institutes of Health (NIH) before returning to the AMC—a fast track to academic stardom sometimes called "the NIH shunt." The single attribute among this elite group, along with ambition and the willingness to work very hard, is that all have mastered academic medicine success skills.

If you are to excel and advance in academic medicine, there are many skills to master. Some—such as negotiation, grant writing, and administration—have been covered in earlier chapters of this book. In this chapter, I will discuss five domains that I think of as success skills. These are taking charge of your career, being mentored, participating in national professional organizations, cultivating good interpersonal relationships, and avoiding fatal career errors.

TAKING CHARGE OF YOUR CAREER

I begin the chapter with this topic—taking charge of your career—because far too many young academic clinicians begin to think about their career trajectories much too late.

I mentioned in Chapter 6 that most academicians write nothing in the first few years on faculty, an example of a prolonged career adolescence in which individuals fail to assume mature, adult responsibility for their futures.

Your Academic Needs Assessment

A good starting point is an academic needs assessment. Table 8.1 helps you identify your attributes and your deficiencies in key skill domains: clinical, teaching, scholarship and research, administration, and success skills in general. Then you go on to develop a faculty development strategic for yourself and plan the steps that need to be taken now on your career advancement path.

Learning to Think like an Academician

If you are to succeed and advance in academic medicine, then you must learn to think like an academician as well as a clinician. Why? When I think of why you and I must adapt to the mindset and values of our academic setting, I think of Hyman Roth's comment to Michael Corleone. It is because, "This is the business we chose." (*The Godfather*, Part II, 1974).

Creativity and Seeing Possibilities

What do we mean by thinking like an academician? Writing in response to an article on Professors Not Professing (JAMA 2004:292:1060–1061), Frank states, ". . . in general, the criteria to be a professor at the university level include demonstration of creativity, ie, the development of some original work of interest to colleagues rather than solely to students. This should be the challenge to the clinician-teacher along the road to academic advancement."[1] The original work may not directly benefit your specific patients, although clinical research on topics such as diabetes management or the optimum care of thromboembolic disease may eventually help patients everywhere.

Academic creativity can mean seeing the *possibilities* in patient care, teaching, and administration. Phototherapy of

TABLE 8.1. Academic needs assessment

I. Domains of Academic Skills
Clinical skills
   What are my current strengths and weaknesses, and what should I do
      now to improve my clinical abilities?

Teaching skills
   What are my current teaching strengths and weaknesses, and what should
      I do now to improve my teaching abilities?

Scholarship and research skills
   What are my current research and scholarship strengths and weaknesses,
      and what should I do now to improve my scholarly abilities?

Administrative skills
   What are my current administrative strengths and weaknesses, and what
      should I do now to improve my abilities as a manager and leader?

Success skills
   What are my current strengths and weaknesses as a faculty member, and
      what should I do now to improve my chances for advancement and
      prepare myself for new roles?

II. Personal Faculty Development Plan
What are three specific things I plan to do in the next year to increase my
   effectiveness as an academician?
   1. _____
   2. _____
   3. _____

III. Progress Toward Career Advancement and Promotion in Rank
After reviewing my curriculum vitae, do I consider myself on track toward
   career advancement and timely promotion to the next rank? If not,
   what needs to be accomplished this year?
   1. _____
   2. _____
   3. _____

---

newborn hyperbilirubinemia began when someone noted a newborn nursery attendant clustering the jaundiced babies by a sunny window because they recovered faster from the jaundice when exposed to light. Might student grades in a first year Introduction to Medicine course predict subsequent performance as an intern? If there is an opening in your department for an associate residency director, might that be the right position for you? Recognizing connections, potential, and opportunities—and having the will to act—brings success in academic medicine.

Professional Socialization

Learning to think like an academician is, in a sense, like learning a new language. Many years ago I worked in France for a few months. I struggled to learn the language, and I felt that a big breakthrough came when one day I realized that I could "think" in French. I believe that the same holds for becoming an academician; you must learn to "think" in academic terms. This intellectual transformation is part of the professional socialization process that we all experience, some successfully and some less so. The process is a shared responsibility between the faculty member and the department leadership, as young academic clinicians learn the importance of collaborating with other faculty members, attending key activities in the greater institution, and networking with colleagues across the nation.

The best department chairs recognize that socialization of each new faculty member is a vital concern for the department and for the institution. Professional socialization can be approached through formal faculty development activities and informally through supportive coaching and progressive increases in responsibilities. Professional socialization is also helped by effective mentoring, which I will discuss shortly.

As one suggestion in learning "academic thinking," I recommend that you read *Academic Medicine*, the journal of the Association of American Medical Colleges.

For example, article titles from a recent issue include "Medical Education as a Process Management Problem" and "Documentation Systems for Educators Seeking Academic Promotion in U.S. Medical Schools." More information is available at www.academicmedicine.org. If you have any doubts about the value of this publication, look at the number of times *Academic Medicine* articles are cited throughout this book.

The Impostor Phenomenon

This book would not be complete without consideration of the *impostor phenomenon*. I first became aware of this occurrence early in my academic career. At a medical school committee meeting, a senior and venerated professor of internal medicine remarked, "We all live in fear that others will discover our level of incompetence." More recently, the daughter of a friend was admitted to Harvard University. The graduate of a public high school, the girl and her parents thought that there must be some mistake, even though she was an honor student. A representative of the admissions office at Harvard shared an observation, "Almost everyone at Harvard feels that they are here by mistake."

The impostor phenomenon occurs when a capable individual feels unqualified for the job he or she currently holds. The feelings can lead to psychological stress and depression. Or perhaps they result in better performance because of the motivation sparked by perceived inadequacy. Certainly considering yourself to be intellectually or clinically less competent than those about you can prevent you from performing your best with comfort.

The impostor phenomenon was first described in women.[2] Later studies showed that it affects both men and women.[3] Students and practitioners of many professions may suffer the impostor syndrome, but I suspect that it is especially common among physicians, especially academic clinicians. If you begin to suspect that you are less capable than those about you and you fear that others will discover your inadequacy, you may be experiencing the impostor phenomenon. Studying the growing body of literature on the topic may help.[4] It may also be time for a conversation with a trusted mentor or advisor.

BEING MENTORED AND MENTORING

When he was president of the Association of American Medical Colleges, Dr. Robert G. Petersdorf wrote, "In my career I have profited enormously from the interactions I have had with those who served as my mentors."[5] Our book's contributors had a lot to say about mentoring. In response to the question, "Have you had a mentor and, if so, how has that person influenced your career?" I received the following responses:

- "I have had a number of influential mentors. Having had no medical or academic role models until after college, linking up with mentors has been vital to my education as an aspiring academic clinician."
- "I had a mentor in fellowship. I have a mentor now, but he lives far away and we only communicate by e-mail and occasionally by phone. He influenced my career by guiding my research. If I am interested in two things and he is interested in only one, then that's what we do, because I know I will need his help."
- "I've had several informal mentors who have helped guide me and warned me about some of the less obvious pitfalls along the way."
- "My mentor helped me understand how to negotiate the system in residencies and in the academic medical center. He also has helped me make important and useful connections with people."
- "Yes, my first chair. He gave me expectations and told me basically to 'go for it.' He also guided me and gently corrected my errors. He told me to dream big dreams."
- "Most of my key decisions were made as a result of mentorship."
- "An important unwritten rule is to know when to leave a mentor in order to branch out in a new direction."
- "Yes, both my former service chiefs were men of great personal integrity and knowledge, who shared their expertise with those who were their students. They always felt as if they were learning more from us than giving to us."
- "Intellectual mentors are hugely important in medicine because so many doctors think alike. It was Alan Kay who said, 'A new point of view is worth 80 IQ points.' Having

the right point of view is critical in academia (and elsewhere). And my administrative mentor, an MD department chair, was just flat-out brilliant when it came to program development and getting things done. It was nice to see that and I always think back on it when I'm doing things."

- ◾ "I think that you can have multiple mentors at one time—using them based on the tasks or needs at hand."

- ◾ "I have had three mentors who have provided me with guidance and have served as role models in various ways. The first taught me about leadership and the use of institutional influence. The second showed me how to use imagination and wonder in the academic world. The third taught me about communities and that the real world is outside of the university."

- ◾ "I must consider my parents first in this category because from them I acquired my desire to ask questions, learn and enrich my life. In my work thus far, I have been fortunate to work with several fine scholars and gentlemen. The ones I admire most are those who manage a healthy mix between their professional and personal lives. I have seen firsthand that having an intellectually satisfying and robust practice while at the same time being a good spouse and parent are not mutually exclusive. It takes extraordinary people to balance their lives well, and I am continually striving to find that sense of balance for myself. I have learned that it can be done."

- ◾ "Identify and choose a mentor who is in the position you wish to achieve in five years. Make sure you have similar values, e.g., 'chemistry.' Learn how to be available at times convenient for the mentor and to follow carefully the milestones that are suggested."

About the Role of Mentors

I hope that the comments above have convinced you of the importance of a mentor in your career. In fact you may have several mentors: one for research, one for your administrative activities, and yet another for your career advancement. Choose your mentors with care. The selection of a mentor may, in retrospect, turn out to be a pivotal career decision.

A mentor must not be selected haphazardly. In a study of mentoring of academic medicine faculty, Jackson and colleagues concluded, "Finding a suitable mentor requires effort and persistence. Effective mentoring necessitates a certain chemistry for an appropriate interpersonal match. Prized mentors have 'clout,' knowledge, and interest in the mentees, and provide both professional and personal support." The researchers did not conclude that same-gender or same-race matches between mentor and mentee were essential.[6]

The mentor serves on several levels. First of all, the mentor is likely to act as a coach, providing guidance in a specific area, such as scholarly activity, and helping the mentee develop a career vision and achieve the goals associated with this vision.[7] He or she may act as a counselor and, for example, would be a likely person to consult if you feel overwhelmed with work or are beginning to feel a little like an impostor. Certainly the mentor will serve as a role model, if only in a domain such as leadership or clinical care. In all cases, the mentor must "place the fellow or junior faculty member's goals above programmatic or institutional goals."[8]

Although mentoring is a two-way street, the initiative must be with you, the young academic clinician. You must seek out the senior person you have chosen to be a prospective mentor. Schedule a time to meet with this person to talk about your research, to ask advice about an administrative decision, or just to discuss your career progress. If the "chemistry" seems to be there, schedule another visit, then another. It is entirely possible that the word "mentor" may never come up in conversation, but the relationship may develop all the same.

In time, and with experience, you may be sought out as a potential mentor. Be receptive to the young faculty member seeking your help and guidance. Being open to acting as a mentor is one way to give something back to the system that helped you. And you may well learn some things in the process.

PROFESSIONAL ORGANIZATIONS

Being active in professional organizations can be a very important part of academic life. Every specialty has its national clinical/political organization that chiefly serves the needs of practicing physicians. Furthermore, these national organizations often have state and, sometimes, local chapters. In addition, for every specialty there are national academic organizations that can be helpful to faculty clinicians. Some of these specialty and academic organizations are listed in Table 8.2.

Within each of these organizations there two options for participation. One is to serve on a committee or task force or even to run for elected office. The other is to become a speaker at an annual meeting, whether on a clinical or a pedagogical topic, or to present the results of a clinical research study. The latter activity is especially beneficial to your career advancement because it allows you to log a research presentation and perhaps an abstract on your curriculum vitae (see Chapter 4). Presenting at national meetings increases your national network of colleagues, allows you to see who is doing what work in your area of specialization, and helps establish your reputation as an expert on your career topic.

I believe that you should select one national organization and direct your efforts there. This lets you become one of the "in group" and affords you the platform to run for elected office if you ever so desire. It helps assure you a spot on the program if you wish to be a speaker. On the other hand, attending a variety of professional society meetings each year seems to assure that you will never achieve leadership in any one of them.

My advice is the same as for mentorship—get started. Select a target organization, whether clinical or academic, early in your career. Then do your best to attend meetings regularly and become an active committee member or program speaker as soon as you can.

TABLE 8.2. Selected specialty and academic societies and organizations that may be pertinent for academicians

Association of American Medical Colleges

Anesthesiology
    Association of University Anesthesiologists
    Society for Education in Anesthesia

Dermatology
    Association of Professors of Dermatology

Emergency Medicine
    Association of Academic Chairs of Emergency Medicine
    Council of Emergency Medicine Residency Directors
    Society for Academic Emergency Medicine

Endocrinology
    Endocrine Society

Family Medicine
    American Academy of Family Physicians
    Association of Departments of Family Medicine
    Association of Family Medicine Residency Directors
    Society of Teachers of Family Medicine

General Surgery
    American Surgical Association
    Association for Academic Surgery
    Association for Surgical Education
    Society of University Surgeons

Immunology
    Training Program Directors of the American Academy of Allergy, Asthma
        & Immunology

Internal Medicine
    American College of Physicians
    American Gastroenterological Association
    American Society of Hematology
    Association of American Physicians
    Association of Professors of Cardiology
    Association of Professors of Medicine
    Society of General Internal Medicine

Multispecialty
    American Geriatrics Society
    American Medical Women's Association

Neurology
    American Academy of Neurology
    American Neurological Association
    Association of University Professors of Neurology

TABLE 8.2. *Continued.*

Neurosurgery
  American Association of Neurological Surgeons
  Society of Neurological Surgeons

Obstetrics and Gynecology
  American College of Obstetricians and Gynecologists
  American Society for Reproductive Medicine
  Association of Professors of Gynecology and Obstetrics

Ophthalmology
  Association of University Professors of Ophthalmology

Orthopaedics
  American Orthopaedic Association

Otolaryngology
  Society of University Otolaryngologists/Head and Neck Surgeons

Pediatrics
  Ambulatory Pediatric Association
  American Pediatric Society
  Society for Pediatric Research

Physical Medicine and Rehabilitation
  American Academy of Physical Medicine and Rehabilitation
  Association of Academic Physiatrists

Plastic Surgery
  American Association of Plastic Surgeons
  Plastic Surgery Educational Foundation
  Plastic Surgery Research Council

Preventive Medicine
  Association of Teachers of Preventive Medicine

Psychiatry
  American Association of Directors of Psychiatric Residency Training
  American Psychiatric Association
  Association of Directors of Medical Student Education in Psychiatry

Psychology
  Association of Medical School Psychologists

Radiology
  Association of University Radiologists

Thoracic Surgery
  American Association for Thoracic Surgery
  Thoracic Surgery Directors Association

Urology
  Society of University Urologists

Vascular Surgery
  Society for Vascular Surgery

INTERPERSONAL SKILLS: PLAYING NICELY IN THE SANDBOX

The career rewards for your hard work and study to learn about excellence in patient care, teaching, and scholarship can be denied if you fail to get along with your colleagues. In order to advance in academia, a faculty member cannot be perceived as selfish, hostile, underhanded, or goofy. You cannot be a curmudgeon or a poor citizen. In the words of grade-school children, "Don't be smart in school and dumb on the bus."

Hogging Resources

A favorite aphorism in academic medicine is, we fight so hard because the stakes are so low. In academia, our salaries are set by negotiation and by our patient care income and perhaps the grants we get. So we generally don't fight about huge sums of money. The battles in academia are often about resources that might seem trivial to our colleagues in the business world: office location, access to administrative assistance, new computers, research space, even where we park. It is right and fair to advocate for your fair share of these treasured resources, but only to a point. If you come to be viewed as a resource hog, your stock in the department will go down.

Turf Wars

In medical academia, there can be vicious battles between specialties for clinical opportunities and curriculum time. In your medical center, has there ever been an issue as to who does head and neck surgery—the otolaryngologists, the plastic surgeons, or another group of surgical specialists? Have the pediatricians and the internists ever disputed your medical center's definition of the age at which pediatric medicine ends and adult medicine begins? Does surgery for herniated lumbar disks belong to the neurosurgeon or the orthopaedic surgeon, or is it shared amicably? What specialty should direct the course that teaches physical diagnosis to medical students?

Turf wars are common in academic medicine. They generally occur at high levels, but not always. The principle to keep in mind is this: I should negotiate very hard for my interests, and I must not be bullied. However in the end, I must maintain a working relationship with my opponent, because tomorrow we may need to work together caring for a patient or teaching a course. An important lesson for young faculty to learn is just how long to battle in a turf war and then when to seek a settlement that all can live with.

Land Mines

Stepping on a land mine can severely damage your career. Land mines are hazards that you might encounter suddenly, unexpectedly, and even innocently, or at least without thinking things through carefully. Here are four land mines for you to avoid carefully.

Harassment

Your professional life is spent in a setting that has rules to protect the individual against unfair treatment. Never act out your frustration with a fellow faculty member in a way that might be construed as harassment. For example, never make disparaging public remarks about a person, do not leave angry notes in his or her mailbox or on the door to the person's office, and do not file frivolous complaints about a person. Be especially careful about anything you write. Even if you have an ongoing reason to be angry with a fellow faculty member, it is best to put your feelings aside and go on with your business—unless there is an unassailable and documentable reason for your grievance.

Discrimination

Be especially careful not to do or say anything that might be seen as biased against anyone based on gender, race, and all the other reasons we know well. This includes one-to-one conversations. In today's political climate, a claim of discrimination can cut short your career if it is substantiated. Even if a claim is spurious, its existence on the record can create problems for you for a very long time.

Plagiarism

Recently I was teaching a writing seminar and we had a guest, a medical editor for a major scientific publisher. I asked this individual what he thought was the biggest problem in medical publishing today. His answer surprised me. He identified the biggest problem as plagiarism. In the world of newspaper and trade publishing (books for the general public), we have recently heard about instances of plagiarism. To be charitable, I believe that some of these instances began as research, often by research assistants, and that eventually the author lost track of the fact that he was actually using someone else's words. I think sometimes this is "accidental plagiarism." However this happens, medical writers must guard vigilantly against even the hint of appropriating intellectual property. This calls for careful documentation of the sources of all bibliographic research and diligent use of citations in the final document to avoid even the appearance of plagiarism.

Scud Missiles

These are angry memos directed at an individual or perhaps a committee composed of individuals. Scud missiles used to be sent as letters or typed memos; now they are launched by e-mail. Be especially wary of sending the Scud missile. It can self-inflict more damage than even a personal attack or an angry outburst at a meeting. Why? Because you have provided future adversaries written documentation of your poor judgment. With a few keystrokes, a recipient of a Scud missile can send your message as an e-mail attachment to everyone on the entire faculty.

FATAL CAREER ERRORS

Harry Truman once said, "Three things can ruin a man, power, money, and women. I never wanted power, I never had money, and the only woman in my life is up at the house right now."[9] I would consider the obsessive pursuit of any of these to be a fatal career error. In academic medicine, there are even more possibilities to bring ruin upon yourself. Fatal career errors represent a series of choices you make that can doom your future, all because you did not pay attention to the law of unintended consequences. Here are some of them.

Fighting the Culture

I have been in academic medicine long enough to see young clinicians join a faculty, neglect to engage in scholarly activity, fail to join institutional committees, avoid social contact with colleagues outside the workplace, and then fail to receive the rewards of academia (notably promotion in rank) and leave in frustration. This scenario is a special risk for primary-care clinicians, who may assume faculty positions believing—falsely—that the academic community will somehow abandon centuries of tradition and promote them solely because they are good clinicians.

Losing Clinical Skills

Teaching demands that you have clinical skills that are up-to-date. The clinician-teacher who loses clinical skills soon loses teaching credibility. Clinicians who become involved in research and administration find that they have less and less patient contact. As "academic" duties increase and clinical duties dwindle, it is entirely possible to work in a major medical center and lose your clinical skills. With absolutely no data to support my assertion, I believe that 30% patient-care time is the absolute minimum needed to maintain clinical skills. If you give up hospital or operating room work, you will lose skills you worked very hard to attain. If you give up a facet of patient care for 2 years or more—attending in the intensive care unit, for example—you are unlikely to resurrect that particular skill.

If your career path has taken you to a clinical research or administrative focus, this may be well and good. But in Chapter 2, I mentioned that your patient-care skills are your job security as a clinician. If you give up your clinical skills for a grant-dependent future in research or begin climbing the administrative ladder and then fall, you may be unable to return to seeing patients for a living.

Going Legal

Going legal can become a way of life for some naïve faculty members. I have seen legalistic tendencies in the person who invokes "rules of order" at an open faculty meeting, citing regulations and bylaws in order to advance a favored cause. Eventually, despite winning some victories, this person becomes universally disliked.

The next level is filing grievances: "Dr. X used my data without asking me." "Dr. Y preempted my operating room time." "Dr. Z gave the lecture that I always give."

The pinnacle of "going legal" is filing formal charges of harassment or discrimination. There is an old saying: He who goes to the law holds a wolf by the tail. If you ever think about filing such a charge, consider very carefully what you are doing. Yes, you may be striking a blow for what you believe to be fairness and equality. Recognize, however, that while you may be punishing someone you believe to be a wrongdoer, you are marking yourself as one who is prepared to deal with problems by formal complaints and even litigation. In the future, those who consider you for a job, a coveted committee appointment, or a leadership position may see your willingness to go to the law as a danger signal. But you will never know.

Betting Your Career Future

At some time in your career, you will be "mad as hell" about a decision and be ready to put your job on the line. I have seen a venerated faculty member quit her job in protest over an issue, and yet most of her colleagues did not know about the issue; they just knew she quit and did not know why. Failure and disappointment are part of any human enterprise. Mature individuals accept this and move on. But some day you may want to say, "If I don't get this promotion, I'm quitting," or "If this teaching program is canceled, I'm leaving." If you take such a confrontational position as your BATNA (best alternative to a negotiated agreement), I suggest that you begin to collect cardboard boxes and start packing your office possessions.

Smart academic clinicians do not make impetuous career moves. Instead they learn effective management of their careers and their lives, which I will discuss in the next chapter.

REFERENCES

1. Frank GW. Letter to the Editor. JAMA 2004;292:2972.
2. Clance P, Imes S. The impostor phenomenon in high-achieving women: dynamics and therapeutic intervention. Psychotherapy: Theory, Research and Practice 1978;15:241–247.
3. Holmes SW, Kertay L, Adamson LB, et al. Measuring the impostor phenomenon: a comparison of Clance's IP Scale and Harvey's IP Scale. J Pers Assess 1993;60:48–59.
4. Harvey JC, Katz C. If I'm so successful why do I feel like a fake: the impostor phenomenon. New York: St. Martin's Press, 1985.
5. Petersdorf RG. Presidential address. Am J Surg 1987; 154:465–469.
6. Jackson VA, Palepu A, Szalacha L, Caswell C, Carr PL, Inui T. Having the right chemistry: a qualitative study of mentoring in academic medicine. Acad Med 2003;78:328–334.
7. Schrubbe KF. Mentorship: a critical component for professional growth and academic success. J Dental Educ 2004; 68:324–328.
8. Applegate W, Williams ME. Career development in academic medicine. Am J Med 1990;88:263–267.
9. Truman HS. Quoted in: Axelrod A. When the buck stops with you: Harry S. Truman on leadership. New York: Penguin Books, 2004.

9

How to Manage Your Career and Your Life

Sir William Osler described "the need for a lifelong progressive personal training."[1] I note that Sir William stated "personal" and not professional or clinical training. Thus, in a broad interpretation, I read the stated need as describing lifelong attention to one's career as a clinician and an academician and the integration of this career with one's life as a human being. Some of the domains to be considered include attention to the life stages in the life of an academic clinician, how to maintain career vitality, and ways to improve your skills as a clinician and an academician throughout your career and your life.

LIFE STAGES IN YOUR CAREER

One of the lessons we learn in life is that what is important to us changes as we grow older and—we hope—wiser. There are changes in our goals, our wants, and our needs. The changes occur according to each individual's confluence of physical aging, emotional maturity, health problems, and even wealth accumulation. The high-excitement, high-stress job that you loved in your thirties can be an enormous burden when in your fifties.

No stage of your career is "better" than another, but each has its characteristics. For purposes of this chapter I have identified five stages in your academic career: contemplative, early career, middle career, late career, and then retirement. I have carefully avoided specifying ages for the various stages described.

Table 9.1 tells your assets and liabilities at the five stages of your academic career. The assets are what you bring to the job as an academic clinician and are why an academic

Table 9.1. Assets and liabilities at five stages of your academic career

Academic career stage	Your assets	Your liabilities
Contemplative stage	Clinical knowledge and skills.	Organizational naiveté.
Early career	Energy and enthusiasm. Willingness to learn new academic skills.	Inexperience in teaching, research, and how to negotiate for needed resources. Tension about role conflicts.
Midcareer	Experience. Awareness of "how the game is played." Self-confidence in academic role.	Conflicting obligations. Held to higher performance standards than before. Concern that career may be hitting a plateau.
Late career	Wisdom and respect. Permission to cut back on activities seen as less fulfilling. More time for thoughtful reflection. Opportunity to develop new areas of expertise.	Declining energy. Concern that abilities are becoming outdated and that career is stagnating.
Retirement	Admiration for your career accomplishments. Financial independence. Time available to contribute as you wish.	The conflicting time demands of retirement activities. Declining health status.

clinical department might hire you or, later, value you as a seasoned veteran.

With each stage in your academic medicine career come developmental milestones. Listed in Table 9.2 are tasks you and I generally must complete in order to reach our maximum potential in a career stage and to prepare to move to the next time of life.

The Contemplative Stage of Your Career

This stage of an academic career represents the time when you are considering and negotiating an academic position.

For most clinicians, this is the late twenties or thirties in age, but because the stage reflects a time of decision about an academic career, it can begin any time that you consider the academic option. For example, one of our contributors decided to leave private practice and enter academic medicine in his late fifties; for him, the contemplative stage began then.

The contemplative stage can be an unsettled time, as you are considering leaving a familiar life—such as residency, fellowship, or practice—and entering an arena that can be quite different from what you have done in the past. In Chapter 3, I described the academic medical center (AMC) value and reward system, which is quite different than other

TABLE 9.2. Developmental tasks at five stages of your academic career

Academic career stage	Chief developmental tasks
Contemplative stage	Learn about academic medical life.
	Avoid biased and bad advice.
	Make the right decision for you.
Early career	Learn the "rules of the game" about the organizational culture.
	Identify a career topic.
	Set limits and avoid overload.
	Find a mentor.
	Consider an academic faculty development fellowship.
Midcareer	Avoid career stagnation.
	Be a mentor for one or more young faculty members.
	Accept more organizational roles in the academic center: committees and task forces, management and leadership activities.
	Become more active in national professional organizations.
Late career	Find new professional challenges.
	Develop a new skill, such as medical writing.
	Lead small-group teaching for medical students.
	Seek opportunities to serve, such as chairing institutional committees and task forces.
	Plan for an active retirement.
Retirement	Select some limited professional activity that will maintain your contact with colleagues.

types of medical practice. In 1978, I decided to leave a very successful solo private practice and enter academic medicine; my parents were dismayed. They asked, "Why in the world are you doing this? Why are you leaving your patients and the practice you have built and moving to something you don't really know anything about?" In retrospect, this was a very good—actually, life-changing—career decision for me, but I wasn't totally sure at the time, and the contemplative stage was, as I think back, a stressful period.

Early Career

This stage begins when you arrive on campus. There is some apprehension about the new challenges, but you know that you are entering an exciting phase of your life. Yes, there will be some role ambiguity and you will often be perplexed by what is expected of you. The conduct of the academic enterprise may seem baffling: How do I accomplish a patient referral in a huge system with students, residents, fellows, and faculty of various ranks? How do I develop a research idea? How do I find a mentor?

When professional basketball player Jason Kidd was first drafted by the Dallas Mavericks in 1994, he exclaimed, "We're going to turn this team around 360 degrees."[2] Like Jason Kidd, you may inadvertently be off the mark at times in your early career. However, because you come with fresh ideas, your early career scholarly work may be the best you ever do. I urge you to look back at Figure 5.2, which shows peaks of academic career productivity; note the early career peak showing work that reflects innovation, enthusiasm, and even fearlessness.

The early career academic clinician will need to learn about performance expectations, how to behave in the academic setting, and the boundaries of what can be accomplished. Can I open a sports medicine clinic if I wish to do so? Can I approach a local foundation for funding to help reduce teen pregnancy? May I make a patient referral directly to the chief of neurosurgery?

There will be a predictable tendency to accept too many opportunities. The newly arrived faculty member will be offered a number of very tempting opportunities—to join a clinical team, participate in a teaching program, or work with a group seeking grant funding for an interesting project. Seasoned faculty members lurk in waiting for young faculty to join their teams and take on the thankless, low-payoff tasks. The latter may be caring for more than your share of "difficult" patients, facilitating small-group teaching of arcane topics, or writing the boring parts of long grants. Because the new faculty member seems to have lots of free time, at least before his or her clinical schedule gets busy, the tendency is to quickly overload your plate.

Your Middle Career

The middle years of an academic career can be a time of maximum productivity or of career stagnation. The choice will be up to you. During the midcareer years you will have the experience that allows you to understand how to get things done in the AMC. Your know-how will also bring you self-confidence and recognition. You will receive valued clinical referrals, hold senior roles on committees, and be invited to join promising scholarly projects. You are likely to be recruited for leadership tasks in your department or in the greater institution. Many midcareer academicians become active in national and even international professional organizations, which offer opportunities for lecturing, consulting, and travel. This is also a time when younger faculty members may seek you out to be their mentors. All in all, the middle years can be the high point of your academic career.

It will also be a time of questioning what you are doing. Am I interested in teaching the Introduction to Clinical Medicine course again for the tenth year in a row? Do I really want to pass a colonoscope five times again today? Does anybody really care about the research I am doing? What is happening in this instance is analogous to a personal midlife crisis, which often comes in the mid-forties and may follow an awareness of having only so many years left before old age and what comes after that. The answer to "hitting a career air-pocket" is to look at fresh opportunities within the context of your current job. These may be learning a new clinical skill, developing an innovative teaching program, or pursuing a fresh research direction.

Your Late Career

In the late career years, often after three decades in academics, you are likely to be recognized as an expert in your field, an authority whose advice is sought and valued. You may be tapped to lead special projects for the institution, task forces and committees that require the prestige of experienced leadership. Young investigators will bring you interesting projects, with invitations to join their research teams and perhaps become "last author" on the final paper. This is clearly a time when you can be a powerful mentor who helps nurture the next generation. In short, if you have been a collaborative and productive academician during the past years, this is a time when good opportunities come to you.

The late career is also a time, like the retirement years to come, to do what you really like to do and stop doing those things that cause stress or that you really don't like to do. Some academic clinicians give up the most physically challenging parts of their practice—delivering babies in the middle of the night, performing the very long surgical procedures, taking night and weekend call, or assuming hospital duties. What you may give up clinically varies with your specialty. You may also give up some time-consuming administrative tasks, such as serving as residency director or department chair.

As you give up some professional activities, you must avoid career stagnation. To do so, many choose to develop new abilities, ideally those that can be continued part-time in retirement. Examples include medical writing, newsletter or journal editing, development (fund-raising) activities, and organizational consulting. Senior faculty status allows you to seek innovation and diversity of professional interests, perhaps attending to intriguing options that younger faculty are too busy to pursue, what Berquist and colleagues call "voices from other rooms."[3]

A key goal of being a senior faculty member is to orchestrate a smooth transition into retirement, leaving with grace at the appropriate time without becoming a *dinosaur*. The academic dinosaur describes an older faculty member who, like his namesake, has failed to adapt and is headed for extinction but fails to recognize these facts. The dinosaur continues to do clinical work after skills have become outdated and teaches by telling tales of past exploits instead of providing evidence-based solutions to clinical problems. If you ever sense that you are heading toward dinosaur status, it is time to consider either retraining or retirement.

Retirement

One of the virtues of academic medicine is that one can transition gradually into retirement. During the senior faculty years you can give up administrative and teaching responsibilities one by one, very gradually, until you are serving a single function such as leading a discussion group for medical students or sitting on a senior administrative committee. One venerated, retired faculty member in our AMC leads a seminar series for senior faculty members. The advantage of retaining some formal official duties is that you remain in contact with the institution, with all its social connections. The continuing interaction with professional colleagues, without a long list of attendant demands or responsibilities, can be very supportive during the retirement years while you enjoy the legacy your career has created.

MAINTAINING CAREER VITALITY

Both community and academic clinicians should be concerned about maintaining career vitality. Being a clinician involves profound responsibilities involving the welfare of patients; becoming an academic clinician can seem to increase the burden, with the addition of teaching and scholarly duties. For some, the diverse challenges of the academic setting are invigorating. For others, they prove to be too much, and the individual may experience career stagnation or burnout.

Career stagnation occurs when a faculty member seems to run out of gas. He or she seems to have no new research questions, has not published a paper in several years, finds ways to avoid clinical care and teaching, and has little to add in administrative meetings. Some call this being "stuck." The curriculum vitae goes out of date, promotion is stalled, and the individual's career is going nowhere. "Stuck" faculty members feel as though others are passing them by, a reality that leads to a loss of self-esteem and confidence.

Burnout occurs when the faculty member becomes implacably frustrated with the job and actively considers some other area of employment; there may be somatic symptoms or evidence of depression. Fatigue and insomnia are common manifestations. A faculty clinician experiencing burnout may be experiencing flagrant career stagnation or actually may appear to be "at the top of his game." What matters in burnout is the individual's response to the stress of the job.

Stagnation and becoming "stuck" may occur during any of the academic career life stages described in Tables 9.1 and 9.2 but are most common midcareer. During your early career, you have enthusiasm and new ideas that can dispel any thought of stagnation. The later career years are a time of consolidating gains and beginning to divest yourself of the more taxing duties. In preserving career vitality, your most vulnerable time is the middle of your career, which, as I noted above, also is the time one is most at-risk for a personal midlife crisis, a temporal relationship that is not a coincidence.

What Influences Job Satisfaction?

In a meta-analysis, Gerrity and colleagues looked at career satisfaction among clinician-educators.[4] They found that the studies examined allowed them to identify seven job characteristics that related to career satisfaction: resources needed for practice, quality of care provided, professional relationships, patient relationships, autonomy, status, and pay. In the specific domain of teaching, the authors note that, "Furthermore, clinician-educators may experience the same intrinsic rewards teaching brings to grade school and high school teachers: the joy of teaching itself and the gratification of witnessing students' mastery of skills and future career successes."

What are the factors that can tip the scales between career satisfaction and vitality versus stagnation or burnout? Demmy and colleagues studied physicians' perceptions of institutional and leadership factors influencing their job satisfaction at a medical center.[5] In the study they included both current faculty and those who had left the institution. The following factors independently predicted good job satisfaction: "Protected time for research or personal use," "equitable distribution of salary/resources," and "trust-communication with chair/division head." Respondents also gave strong consideration to the quality of life in the local community, intellectual issues, and humanitarian issues. Noteworthy, in my opinion, were responses given why faculty would consider opportunities elsewhere: administrative frustration, income enhancement, career advancement, academic frustration, improve research, physician support, clinical programs, and autonomy.

At this point, the astute reader will be thinking that almost all of the issues identified in the Demmy and colleagues study are institutional and not personal (i.e., not under control of the individual faculty member). This is fundamentally true, but also consider that all faculty face at least administrative frustrations, all would like their incomes enhanced, all would like to be promoted, and so forth. What is under your control is your emotional reaction to the stresses we all face.

As one of our contributors reported, "Academic medicine is, somewhat, still a solo career option as the expertise one holds in a subspecialty arena usually will not be held by another individual at the same institution. Thus, collaboration is often at a national or international level. Thus, as it is a solo endeavor at many times, one must believe in one's abilities, keep pushing forward and never let others detract from the course. The limit is set by the individual, not the collective."

Maintaining Job Satisfaction and Career Vitality in Academic Medicine

According to Bland and Berquist, "Faculty vitality is best preserved through preventive measures rather than heroic measures to save "stagnant" or "stuck" faculty.[6] Maintaining career vitality is—or should be—a shared responsibility of the individual academic clinician and the academic medical center, the latter generally represented by his or her clinical department. The best clinical department chairs assure an ongoing program of faculty enrichment, which may include faculty development programs and perhaps access to teaching or research fellowships, described below. Many departments, however, do not offer these opportunities, and the academic clinician must develop his or her own strategy to avoid career stagnation or burnout. Your department's ongoing faculty enrichment program or your own career vitality maintenance plan may include one or more of the following. If not, I urge you to investigate them on your own.

Sabbaticals

If you have the good fortune to work at an AMC that has sabbaticals available, I recommend that you consider the option. Before doing so, of course, you must prepare a sabbatical proposal with the same diligence that you would write a research protocol or grant proposal. Your sabbatical proposal should include:

- What you wish to accomplish during your sabbatical.
- Why this goal cannot be accomplished at our own institution and instead necessitates your spending the time in Paris or Nepal.
- What funding you will need, why each requested item is needed, and where you will find the money.
- How your study or work during the sabbatical will benefit your institution upon your return.

Mini-sabbaticals

Some departments allow "mini-sabbaticals." These are departmentally supported short blocks of time off that allow a faculty member to complete a grant proposal or write up a paper for publication. In short, the department's clinical faculty members all agree that you may have a week or even two free to complete a scholarly task. Your income will continue and your patient care will be covered. Generally, the department chair and/or a small governing committee administer the program.

The philosophy behind the mini-sabbatical is the reciprocity norm (see Chapter 7) in action. I will cover your week off to finish your paper now, and in exchange I expect that you will do so for me—or someone else—at some time in the future. This concept holds that if I do you a favor, I can expect one in return—from you or even from someone else.[7] To study the reciprocity norm, a researcher sent Christmas cards to a group of people he did not know. Most sent back a card and some added the researcher's name to their permanent Christmas card list.[8] Much of what we do in academic medicine is based on the reciprocity norm.

Reinventing Yourself Administratively

Many in academic medicine find that they have undergone one or more such personal reinventions. A major course correction, of course, would be a move from private practice to academic medicine. Once inside the AMC, career stagnation or burnout can be avoided by changing jobs within the department. For example, a faculty colleague with a rural patient-care background became interested in clinical research; he reinvented himself as leader of a rural practice–based research network.

Changing administrative roles within a department is a good way to make a midcourse career change. A clinic director can become residency director. An educator with management skills can become a departmental predoctoral director. Virtually all institutional committees require committed leaders.

Career Rejuvenation Through Medical Writing and Editing

Another way to reinvent your self and maintain career vitality is through medical writing and editing. Although this may seem especially attractive to senior faculty, it is available to academic clinicians at any stage of professional life. By medical writing and editing, I am not referring to writing reports of clinical research for publication in peer-reviewed journals; we should all do this. Instead, your daily activities will gain new meaning when you write about them, perhaps as a "Day in the Life" column for a medical publication, as poetry, or as a fictionalized story. Consider writing or editing a reference book in your specialty; you may begin by writing chapters for books edited by others, until you learn the system. Getting the invitation to write or edit a medical reference book is easier than most might think.[9]

If writing or editing a book seems too ambitious, you might consider writing review articles for advertiser-supported journals, editing a medical newsletter, or joining the editorial board of a journal. These opportunities, as with writing or editing a medical book, are often possible, if only you make the inquiry.

At some institutions there are even short programs to promote writing skills. One program described is the Scholarly Writing in Academic Medicine Program embedded in a Collaborative Mentoring Program (CMP). The writing portion consists of seven 75-minute sessions covering various aspects of medical writing.[10] The CMP program is representative of the types of programs that individual clinical departments can present on any of a variety of topics.

I have emphasized medical writing and editing as a means of avoiding career stagnation and burnout for several reasons. First of all, writing is a natural adjunct to medical care and teaching and is something you can do on your own schedule, with few resources other than your computer, and in the odd bits of time available to you. Writing can help you develop new perspectives to otherwise mundane events in your life. It brings valuable and enriching professional networking and can help your eventual candidacy for promotion. Writing also happens to be my favorite hobby.

Community Service and Career Vitality

For the clinician in academic medicine, a logical way to prevent or overcome career stagnation is through community service. The academic clinician can volunteer to work in a clinic for the homeless. Another, more ambitious, option is to initiate such a clinic, helping medical students and residents gain patient-care experience and serve their community. An adventurous approach to maintaining career vitality is to take time off to serve the needy in a developing country.

Other Ways to Maintain Career Vitality

Some faculty members develop innovative programs within the institution; examples include "Literature and Medicine" or "Medical History" study groups. For others, career energy can flow from becoming active in a national professional organization. Yet another possibility is speaking to high school and college groups about health topics.

Of course, a classic method of re-energizing your career, and one involving a major time commitment, is the faculty development (FD) fellowship.

FACULTY DEVELOPMENT PROGRAMS, WORKSHOPS, AND FELLOWSHIPS

When asked what advice they would give the new academic clinician, several contributors recommended, "Take a faculty development fellowship." (For the full list of contributors' answers to the "advice to new faculty members" question, see Chapter 10.)

Hamilton and Brown define faculty development as "an organized, goal-directed process to achieve career progression and growth. Inherent in this process is the acquisition of skills that enable one to contribute in a meaningful way to the advancement of a field of interest, whether educational, operational, or scientific."[11] As with any professional endeavor, faculty development involves attitudes, knowledge, and skills. FD activities include programs at a single institution, workshops that have participants from more than one institution, and fellowships.

Faculty Development Programs at the Academic Medical Center

Faculty development programs at your AMC may cover any of a variety of topics: research skills, grant writing, bedside teaching, how to present a lecture, curriculum design, and many of the topics covered in this book. Such programs, which rely on internal talent, are inexpensive for departments to present and are very helpful for young faculty members.

Above I mentioned the writing component of a Collaborative Mentoring Program held in a single medical school. Pololi and colleagues describe their full FD program, which, in addition to scholarly writing, includes key skills for career development and a structured values-based approach to career planning, all based on Rogerian and adult learning principles.[12] Their paper reports that key meaningful outcomes for most participants were identifying their core values, formulating career plans based on these values, developing collaborative relationships, and improving their skills in regard to gender and power issues, negotiation and conflict management, scholarly writing, and oral presentation. Notably in regard to maintaining career vitality, participants in the program reported improved satisfaction in their decisions to remain in academic medicine.

The Medical Education Scholars Program (MESP) at the University of Michigan Medical School aims to develop leaders in medical education, using a competitive selection process and one-half-day per week release time for the 1-year program. Gruppen and colleagues report "measurable impacts on the careers of the participants and the institutional environment."[13]

Workshops

Workshops come in many varieties. All involve a block of time away from one's usual duties and are devoted to gaining knowledge and skills in a focused area. The time commitment may be a half-day, a week, or a month. Many workshops are held at national professional meetings, where you can attend a workshop on flexible sigmoidoscopy, management of coronary heart disease, or finding balance in your life.

Focused workshop topics span the full spectrum of faculty development, including everything you and I can imagine in regard to clinical care, teaching, and scholarship. For example, Pandachuck and colleagues describe a 2-day workshop to improve teaching skills.[14] According to the authors, "The participants uniformly regarded the workshops as helpful" and described the short teaching exercise as the most important component of the program.

Because short-term workshops involve time away from work and home, there is a cost involved. However, the respite from usual duties can be a big plus in maintaining career vitality. This is not to diminish the value of the experience. For example, in a study to assess the long-term effects of a professional development program on physician educators, Armstrong and colleagues surveyed participants in the Harvard Macy Program for Physician Educators 2 years after their participation.[15] In their conclusions, the authors suggest that "professional development programs that create an immersion experience designed in a high-challenge, high-support environment, emphasizing experiential and participatory activities can change behaviors in significant ways, and that these changes endure over time."

Clinical Scholar Programs

The prototype of the ongoing multisite faculty development program is the Robert Wood Johnson (RWJ) Clinical Scholars Program, "designed to augment a physician's clinical training by providing new skills and perspectives necessary to achieve leadership positions both within and outside the walls of academia in the 21st century." The program's latest iteration emphasizes community-based research and leadership training. Currently, four U.S. academic medical centers train participants in the program: University of California, Los Angeles; University of Michigan; University of Pennsylvania; and Yale University. Twenty new positions are funded annually through the RWJ Foundation. The U.S.

Department of Veterans Affairs supports eight additional positions each year through the VA Medical Centers affiliated with the participating AMCs.[16] Information about the RWJ clinical scholars program should be available through your dean's office or at the Web site in Ref. 16.

Research Training Opportunities

The National Institutes of Health offers a wide variety of training opportunities. For full information go to the following Web site: http://www.training.nih.gov/.

Other Possibilities

An option available to clinicians who want to augment pedagogical skills is direct observation or videotaping of teaching activities, reviewed with senior faculty. Although this method may require your initiative, it should be available in any clinical academic department. Some AMCs offer simulated ambulatory teaching situations using "standardized students," analogous to teaching with "standardized patients" (i.e., actors). Lesky and colleagues describe one such program.[17]

The Stanford Faculty Development Program: Professionalism in Contemporary Practice program is a "month-long facilitator-training course that prepares participating faculty to deliver a faculty development curriculum for colleagues and residents at their home site."[18]

Fellowships

A faculty development fellowship is the high-commitment, high-payoff option. These are available in most specialties, and a few are interdisciplinary. Many aspiring young faculty take faculty development fellowships directly after finishing their residency or subspecialty fellowship, although it may be possible to return to a faculty development fellowship during your early career years. This return-to-fellowship option is especially reasonable if you are thinking about a

TABLE 9.3   Faculty development fellowships: representative programs

---

Full-Time
Surgery Education Fellowship, NYU School of Medicine
  This is a "funded one-year position for a resident in surgery or a recent
    graduate of a surgical residency interested in pursuing a career in
    surgical education. The fellowship program will educate fellows in the
    core knowledge and skills of research, teaching and leadership."
Information is available at http://www.facs.org/education/fellowship/html/.

Part-Time
National/Regional Programs
OMERAD (Office of Medical Education Research and Development)
    Primary Care Faculty Development Fellowship Program
  Fellows in this program participate in a 72-day "on campus/at home"
    experience. The campus is the Michigan State University College of
    Human Medicine. The program includes up to 20 participants from
    family medicine, general internal medicine, and general pediatrics. Topics
    covered include "clinical teaching/evaluation, research, administration and
    management, computer skills, written communication, and academic
    socialization."
Information is available at http://www.omerad.msu.edu/fellowship/.

---

part-time commitment. Table 9.3 describes a few representative full-time and part-time fellowships.

You can learn about some faculty development options in your specialty by searching Google: "faculty development fellowships (your specialty)." Your AMC's office of graduate education and your national specialty organization can also provide information.

Faculty development fellowships can give you very useful teaching skills and academic experience. The fellowship also gives you a good start on your national networking. If you are a young clinician thinking about academics or if you are early in your academic career, I recommend that you think seriously about taking a faculty development fellowship.

WHAT OUR CONTRIBUTORS MIGHT DO DIFFERENTLY IF THEY COULD DO IT OVER AGAIN

At this point in the chapter, after considerable discussion about managing your career and your life, I want to share how our contributors responded to the question: "If you could do one thing differently in your career, what would it be?"

- "Devote more time to writing and to understanding statistics. Both skills are needed with writing grants and publications."
- "I would try to spend more time with my family—this is the constant struggle I deal with."
- "I would probably have given more attention to my personal health (exercise, diet) and spent more time with my family."
- "Really learn the basics of clinical research and writing earlier."
- "I wouldn't do anything differently. Everyone can think of moments they would like to do over, such as studying more for an exam or answering an interview question a certain way, but these shrink to insignificance in the big-picture view. The major professional decisions I have made were made after a great deal of reflection, and the results of those decisions have opened my life to opportunities I might otherwise have never encountered."
- "I would have gotten a PhD in biostatistics when I was younger."
- "Explore other interests in college academically in subjects outside medicine and science. That would have helped build a foundation for advancement later in life."
- "I would have spent less time in practice before switching to academics. I was in practice for 13 years."
- "Major in fine arts in college."
- "Start to write early. I didn't do it and now feel I am too old to start."
- "I would have done more research as an assistant professor and learned how to get funding for this."
- "I would have strengthened my research skills to do more high-level scholarly work. I would have not entered administrative positions as early, but would have run more meaningful projects first. The best work is done by project directors."
- "Get fellowship trained."

■ "Other than marry my wife one year earlier (it made the first year of medical school very hard commuting), there are no changes that in retrospect would have provided any greater satisfaction."

In reading over the answers of our contributors, I notice that most of them are very happy with their career decisions. Wishing they had learned more academic skills earlier in their careers was reported commonly. Also, note that several chose to tell about their personal lives.

OTHER CAREER CONSIDERATIONS

I will finish this chapter by discussing some odds and ends about managing your career and your life—items that don't seem to fit under other categories.

Ethical Issues in Academic Medicine

Academic medical centers train tomorrow's physicians, and hence there should be no place for even the hint of unethical behavior—no curriculum vitae inflation, no painted laboratory mice or "fudging" of research data, no grading students on any criteria other than their academic and clinical performance, and no borrowing the ideas of others without permission and attribution.

CV Inflation

In Chapter 4, I discussed how to prepare a CV. Here I will return to the CV to discuss one focused ethical issue: inflation of accomplishments to "puff up" your résumé. In discussing grants written by a team, it is all too easy to write the CV entry to look as though you were the lead or even the sole author. The author list on a published paper is easy to confirm but more difficult to verify for a grant submitted in the past. Even if you are tempted to step into murky ethical waters in listing grant authorship on your CV, remember that the academic community is much smaller than you would ever imagine, and there is considerable institutional memory of who did what on which project.

Recently, I encountered an especially nefarious CV inflation ploy. In 2004, I chaired the scientific program committee for a major international scientific meeting. Our committee was very gratified with the large number of research papers and posters submitted, and we planned our program based on these submissions. Imagine our dismay when many of the presenters for the accepted papers and posters—some with as many as six or eight co-authors—failed to register and attend the meeting. I learned from a colleague in Greece that this happens in international meetings. The no-show presenters know that, by gaining acceptance of their submission, they will be listed as authors in the meeting's abstract book, which they then list as a publication on their CVs. They then see no need to pay for travel costs and meeting registration fees; they have what they wanted—a listed publication. My colleague called these purposefully absent submitters "grasshoppers"—a metaphor that strikes me as appropriate.

The Quest for Any Reportable Result

None of us would think of publishing flagrantly false research findings, but some are tempted to search accumulated data to find a significant P-value somewhere, anywhere. In an intervention that seemed to show no statistical significance, perhaps we will get a different "result" if we examine only subjects under age 50, or perhaps postmenopausal women or married men. This type of data mining is discussed in Chapter 6.

Issues in Reporting of Sponsored Research

A more subtle type of spurious research reporting occurs with sponsored research, when statistically significant results are discussed in a biased way or not published at all. When a pharmaceutical company underwrites research costs, that firm has a vested interest in the outcome and in what is eventually published. The author may feel pressure to write the conclusion in a certain way, especially when the pharmaceutical company offers the authors "editorial assistance" in preparing the research report. And what if the study shows that the drug is no better than placebo? I think that in such an instance, the pharmaceutical company might prefer that results not be published. Yet, the study was done and there was a statistically significant outcome, even if the study drug was not as effective as the control.

The scientific research community has finally recognized the problem and is taking action: "The ICMJE [International Committee of Medical Journal Editors] will require, as a condition of consideration for publication, registration in a public trials registry. Trials must register at or before the onset of patient enrollment. The policy applies to any clinical trial starting enrollment after July 1, 2005."[19]

Academic Evaluation Bias

Would you believe that respected academicians might grade students or residents based on nonacademic criteria? Could it be that educators might select residents for their training programs for reasons that have nothing to do with how good a physician the applicant will be? Yes, these situations occur, and you won't be in academic medicine long before you become aware of how subtle bias becomes involved in the "evaluation" of learners or sometimes of applicants.

We are all familiar with bias based on race, gender, age, and so forth. Academics adds a few more: career choice bias and political bias. As I mentioned in Chapter 1, we all like to "clone" ourselves, and at some medical schools a student on—for example—an internal medicine clerkship might receive a higher final grade than another student who reveals career plans to be a surgeon, psychiatrist, or family physician. Woolley and colleagues found that students, when asked about their career plans, "perceived that their responses could significantly influence the quality of teaching relationships, access to clinical opportunities, and grades."[20]

There are other types of bias. America has become increasingly polarized politically between the so-called conservatives and liberals; you may use different words, but I suspect that you know what I mean. In academia, clerkship final grades and acceptance decisions for medical school or residency are sometimes influenced by the faculty member's opinion of the student's or applicant's political views on topics such as abortion, homosexuality, or even who occupies the White House in Washington, DC. I consider this type of evaluation bias to be academic malpractice, but I am sorry to report that it occurs.

Borrowing Ideas without Permission

Plagiarism, including accidental plagiarism, is discussed in Chapter 8, but there are more subtle forms of unethical borrowing of other persons' intellectual property.

One of the hallmark activities of academic life is meetings, times when very bright people exchange innovative ideas. Often one of these ideas resonates with you, and perhaps it comes to mind later, even at a time weeks later. You write up a research protocol, a grant proposal, or course element. In your enthusiasm, you forget that the idea came from a specific colleague, who suggested it to the meeting group, and that the group had promptly gone on to another topic. You may not recall who first originated the idea, but the author probably will remember and may consider your use of his or her brainchild to be questionable behavior.

Ten years ago, when I lectured at national meetings, I used my 35-mm slides with a short printed handout. Today I use PowerPoint presentations, and my handout is often a printout of my slides, a practice that saves me preparing a separate handout document. With the full text of the speaker's slides in the conference notes, I wonder how many persons subsequently duplicate the slide content and tables and use these in their own lectures. Is this ethical behavior? After all, the PowerPoint slides are not "published" in the sense of being an article or book. Actually they are protected under the copyright law of the United States.[21] But didn't the speaker want us to use the information to teach students, residents, and professional colleagues? Yes, but the speaker almost certainly did not give permission to use his or her specific PowerPoint presentation, and to do so without permission is not ethical behavior.

Academic Personality Disorders

Some of the following certainly occur in industry and commerce and are not unique to academic medicine. Nevertheless, as we consider managing your career and your life, I think it useful to discuss four academic personality disorders.

Perfectionism
Medical academia is a breeding ground for perfectionists. It is so easy to continue tweaking research data, massaging a clinical report, or trudging from committee to committee seeking the flawless version of a program proposal.

Avoid perfectionism by setting personal deadlines and by learning the skill of declaring a project done and launching it into action. If your brainchild is good and it succeeds, great. If there is a problem, you will learn about it soon enough.

Workaholism
Academic medicine also fosters workaholism. Curiously, the excessively long hours and intense effort are often not rewarded financially, as they are in the "piece-work" of private practice, where the more patients you see, the more your earn. Faculty salary base support and faculty practice plans often serve to even out the earnings in a clinical department. Instead, the workaholic toils for the sake of hard work. Perhaps he or she is battling the impostor phenomenon, described in Chapter 8. Maybe there is an inappropriate fear of failure or the delusion of being indispensable, the latter a common affliction of physicians in all specialties. Or maybe you have nothing else in your life other than work, a sad situation that merits urgent attention.

If you are a faculty member and you seldom get home for dinner, have a weekend free of work, or have not had an out-of-town true vacation (not a medical meeting) in a year, then you are probably an academic workaholic.

Helpaholism
One of our contributors writes, "Helping colleagues does not diminish one's own opportunities. In fact, it probably helps." But there is a limit. The helpaholic can't say, "No." This person puts everything aside any time a colleague asks that

a paper be critiqued, a grant proposal be proofread, or a seminar be led. The helpaholic seems to wear a bright label that says, "Take advantage of me!"

To avoid becoming an abused helpaholic, you must learn to prioritize work, remembering that in Chapter 7, I urge you to do your own work first. Develop the skill of delegating to your administrative staff and be aware when they are passing their work to you—upward delegation in the administrative hierarchy. When tasks are assigned at a meeting, resist the urge to volunteer for much more than your share, and be careful that assignments are distributed equitably. In short, stand up tall and stop being a doormat for others.

Disorganization

The academic environment, with its many and diverse opportunities, invites intellectual scatter. The early phase of this academic personality disorder occurs when you say, "yes" to far too many attractive offers. The next stage is subliminal awareness that you cannot complete key projects adequately and on time. You flit from project to project, dithering about details, until your mind winds into a fugue state in which the simplest task seems too much.

Avoid professional disorganization by limiting the obligations that you undertake, completing them on time by using effective personal time-management skills, and avoiding overcommitment as carefully as you would steer clear of contracting a contagious disease.

Integrating Work and Play

What I write next will resonate with some readers and not with others. When I discuss integrating work and play in one's life during lectures, I spy some attendees nodding in agreement while other roll their eyes.

I look at academic medicine as so much fun that I have always felt a little guilty receiving a paycheck every month. I think of my work as play. I take work back and forth between my desk in the office and my desk at home without much regard for where and when things happen. My wife and I entertain medical students and residents for dinner in our home. Our professional colleagues are our friends (Yes, we also have "non-medical" friends.) I don't think that my wife, who is also a faculty colleague, and I are workaholics; we take plenty of time off, spend a lot of days with grand-children, and go on regular vacations. However, I do think that we live the concept of: Turn your work into play, then play hard.

Learning More About How to Manage Your Career and Your Life

You are likely to be at greater risk of mismanaging your career and your life than you are making a major clinical blunder because you lack medical knowledge and skills. I urge you to spend time learning how to adapt to the stages of professional life, maintain career vitality, and understand the personal issues you will face as an academic clinician. Some useful articles, books, and Web sites are presented in Table 9.4.

Table 9.4. Where to learn more about how to manage your career and your life

Articles and books

Bland CJ, Schmitz CC, Stritter FT, Henry RC, Aluise JJ. Successful faculty in academic medicine: essential skills and how to acquire them. New York: Springer, 1990.

Bowman MA, Frank E, Allan DI. Women in medicine: career and life management, 3rd ed. New York: Springer Verlag, 2002.

Skeff KM, Stratos A, Mygdal T, et al. Faculty development: a resource for clinical teachers. J Gen Int Med 1997;12(Suppl 2): S56–S63.

Whitman N. Notes of a medical educator. Salt Lake City: University of Utah, 1999.

Web sites

American College of Physicians: Fellowships and academic medicine. Available at http://www.acponline.org/srf/res_fam.htm/.

Association of American Medical Colleges, selected bibliography, faculty development. Available at http://www.aamc.org/members/facultyaffairs/bibliography/developmentms.pdf/.

Carr PL, Bickel J, Inui J. Taking root in a forest clearing: a resource guide for medical faculty. Available at http://www.bumc.bu.edu/Dept/content.aspx?PageID=8849&departmentid=42/.

Medical forum. Available at http.medicalforum.com/.

REFERENCES

1. Osler W. Quoted in: Breedlove C, ed. Osleriana. JAMA 1986;256:3481–3483.
2. Celebrities. GoofUps.com. Available at http://www.goofups.com/quotes/107_84.html.
3. Berquist WH, Greenburg EM, Klaum GA. In our fifties: voices of men and women reinventing their lives. San Francisco: Jossey-Bass, 1993.
4. Gerrity MS, Pathman DE, Linzer M, et al. Career satisfaction and clinician-educators. J Gen Int Med 1997;12(Suppl. 2): S90–S97.
5. Demmy TL, Kivlahan C, Stone TT, Teague L, Sapienza P. Physicians' perceptions of institutional and leadership factors influencing their job satisfaction at one academic medical center. Acad Med 2002;77:1235–1240.
6. Bland CJ, Berquist WH. The vitality of senior faculty members: snow on the roof—fire in the furnace. Washington DC: ASHE-ERIC Higher Education Report, Vol. 25, No. 7, 1997, p. 83.
7. Cialdini R. Influence: science and practice. New York: Harper Collins, 1993.
8. Reciprocity norm research. ChangingMinds.org. Available at http://www.changingminds.org/.
9. Taylor RB. Writing book chapters and books. In: The clinician's guide to medical writing. Taylor RB, ed. New York: Springer-Verlag, 2005, pp. 167–194.
10. Pololi L, Knight S, Dunn K. Facilitating scholarly writing in academic medicine: lessons learned from a collaborative peer mentoring program. J Gen Int Med 2004;19:64–69.
11. Hamilton GC, Brown JE. Faculty development: what is faculty development? Acad Med 2003;10:1334–1336.
12. Pololi LH, Knight SM, Dennis K, Frankel RM. Helping medical school faculty realize their dreams: an innovative, collaborative mentoring program. Acad Med 2002;77:377–384.
13. Gruppen LD, Frohn AZ, Anderson RM, Lowe KD. Faculty development for educational leadership and scholarship. Acad Med 2003;78:137–141.
14. Pandachuck K, Harley D, Cook D. Effectiveness of a brief workshop designed to improve teaching performance at the University of Alberta. Acad Med 2004;79:798–804.
15. Armstrong EG, Doyle J, Bennett NJ. Transformative professional development of physicians as educators: assessment of a model. Acad Med 2003;78:702–708.

16. The Robert Wood Johnson Scholars Program. Available at http://www.rwjcsp.Stanford.edu/.
17. Lesky LG, Wilkerson L. Using "standardized students" to teach a learner-centered approach to ambulatory teaching. Acad Med 1994;69:955–957.
18. The Stanford Faculty Development Program. Available at http://sfdc.Stanford.edu/.
19. DeAngelis CD, Drazen JM, Frizelle FA, et al. Clinical trial registration: a statement from the International Committee of Medical Journal Editors. JAMA 2004;292:1363–1364.
20. Woolley DC, Moser SE, Davis NL, Bonaminio GA, Paolo AM. Treatment of medical students based on their stated career interests. Teaching and Learning in Medicine 2003;15(3): 156–162.
21. Copyright law of the United States. Available at http://www.copyright.gov/.

10
Planning for the Future

In the past 9 chapters, I have discussed important facts and strategies you need to know to succeed in academic medicine, and because none of the preceding discussions are exhaustive, I have provided lists of articles, books, Web sites, and organizations where you can learn more. If you have assimilated what has been presented so far, and if you have consulted some of the recommended sources, you know more than most early-career academicians and probably more than some in their mid or late careers.

This last chapter is intended to help you plan for your future in academic medicine. In the pages that follow, I will tell our contributors' responses to a question regarding the advice they would give to a new academic clinician and their replies when asked to tell their favorite anecdote about their academic careers. In addition, I don't think the book would be complete without some thoughts about generational issues, the future of academic medicine, and a few modest prognostications based on current events and the comments of experts.

I will offer specific targeted advice—what to do now—for each of the book's intended readers: students, residents, and fellows thinking about possible careers in academic medicine, practicing clinicians considering a major job change to a faculty role, and academic clinicians early in their careers who have discovered that they have much to learn about medical academia.

The last section of this chapter is a personal indulgence: some "rules" that describe success strategies for the academic clinician. These represent a distillation of what to do, and what not to do, selected from what has been discussed in the first 9 chapters, and based on the responses of our contributors and my own 27-year adventure in academic medicine.

ADVICE FROM THOSE WHO HAVE WALKED THE TRAIL

At the very beginning of this book, you will find the old proverb attributed to an unknown and long-departed Chinese philosopher: If you want to know what lies ahead on the trail, ask someone who has made the journey and returned. I have lived in Oregon since 1984—an "Oregonian by choice." As I read books about the great Oregon Migration in the mid-1800s, I learned that after the first pioneer trailblazers made the journey, scouts who knew where to find water and where there might be danger guided later wagon trains. Later there were even Oregon Trail "road maps" of sorts, recorded by those whose who had made the journey and returned.

In the spirit of asking those who have walked the trail, I asked our contributors, "What advice would you give to a new academic clinician?" Their responses are listed below. The alert reader will note that there are more responses than contributors to the book. That is because there was a robust and generous outpouring of advice, and a number of contributors offered several suggestions. Even if two or more contributors made the same suggestion, I included all, just to show how respondents agree on some important topics. As you read the following comments, presented in random order, you will note some themes.

- "Get fellowship training."
- "Find mentors" (see Chapter 9).
- "Decide what job you want in 10 years. Then do everything needed to achieve that goal."
- "Hang on to your clinical skills. With all the meetings, research, and classroom teaching, it's easy to see your clinical skills slip away."
- "If entering academics or changing jobs from one institution to another, look for a department where you can do what you are trained to do and want to do, whether it is student teaching, resident training, clinical research, or health policy work."
- "When looking at an academic opportunity, ask if faculty roles are 'locked in' or if faculty can shift comfortably

from one role to another as interests change and skills develop."

- "Go to the university social functions: the welcome dinner for new faculty, the holiday party, the graduation activities. Be an active member of the academic community. This is really part of the job."
- "Get as much clinical experience as you can early in your career. It is the foundation of what you teach."
- "Volunteer for one or two institutional committees—the institutional review board (IRB) is a good one. You will make valuable connections and you will learn a lot that you wouldn't learn by 'staying home' in your own department."
- "Find a mentor to help you learn some of the 'unwritten rules'" (see Chapter 3).
- "Spend some of your career in full-time practice—preferably prior to starting academics, because personal knowledge and credibility will be enhanced."
- "Don't volunteer for too many committees and activities too early."
- "Find out what is important to your boss (department, division, or section chair), and do your best to make him or her successful while at the same time trying to pursue your own interests."
- "Complete a faculty development fellowship."
- "Find a faculty mentor and work closely with this mentor on a project, such as a research study or curriculum plan."
- "For better or worse, medicine is not the most flexible of career choices, and can be very unforgiving to those who change their minds in midstream about career direction. I changed specialties, and my road became a very difficult one in the short term while I found a new path. What you must keep in mind (and what I learned after much frustration) is that when you close some doors, others inevitably open if you are resourceful, diligent, conscientious, and honest."
- "Get to know yourself."
- "If you are new to an academic career, give it at least a 2-year try before giving up."

- "Learn to collaborate. For many physicians, myself included, teamwork does not come entirely naturally. I, for example, am most comfortable relying on and trusting my own intellect and effort. Well, just as no clinician can meet all the medical needs of all patients, academic endeavors will be most sustainable when pursued in the context of a collaborative team approach."

- "Follow through on what you begin, and never commit to anything you cannot complete with excellence and on time."

- "Always be available by some form of communication—electronic media, cell phone, or pager."

- "The advice depends on the choice between a clinical or research track. If going from practice to academics, do a fellowship (preferably 2 years) first. Otherwise the research part of the job will be very difficult."

- "Understand the unwritten rules and your place in the hierarchy."

- "Enjoy the work that you do, and make sure that your interests and needs are met. There are many options; make sure that you explore them. And always think outside the box."

- "Try everything, including some research, before settling down to an academic focus. I think most academic physicians eventually find areas or questions without clear answers. Even if research is not your primary focus, being able to define and refine a research question will enable one to collaborate effectively with colleagues with more research time and experience. Develop personnel and financial management skills along the way."

- "Get trained; get a fellowship or master's degree."

- "Protect your time up front—saying 'no, thanks' can be healthy. Then have a clear idea of what you want for your first big project(s)."

- "Life isn't a dress rehearsal; you only go around once."

- "Be prepared to work hard and communicate broadly."

- "Be honest, have high integrity, and do not betray loyalties. Whatever you say gets around quickly. A private practice may be a 'black box' in regard to privacy. Academia is a 'fish bowl.'"

- "Be a positive person and help others as much as possible. When needs arise, be willing to fill in without getting your plate too full."

- "Identify and choose a mentor who is in the position you wish to achieve in five years. Make sure you have similar values, for example, 'chemistry.' Learn how to be available at times convenient for the mentor and to follow carefully the milestones that are suggested."

- "Be willing to work very hard to get funding, and don't quit applying for grants. In fact, don't quit, period. Most important—you are good enough."

- "Credibility is a very fragile commodity that once lost or compromised is very hard to replace."

- "Be loyal to your supervisors and have them see you as someone who is 'on their bus.'"

- "Don't take yourself too seriously; no one else does."

- "Get protected time to write grant proposals, get money, do research, and publish. Be aware of the seduction of clinical care, which is an enormous amount of fun and provides tons of instant gratification and feedback."

- "Find four hours a week to devote to academic pursuits separate from clinical pursuits. If need be, work on Saturdays or Sundays. Success will not happen unless you are prepared to work regularly and consistently."

- "Start off slowly. Don't commit to too many things early on. Allow yourself some time to test the waters."

- "In academia, the right thing may be done for the wrong reasons. Do not get 'hung up' on the reasons. Academic institutions are driven by money and reputation, yet often do well for society. Don't let yourself get bothered by the sometimes-selfish motivation."

- "Pursue those things that interest you the most, even if you don't understand why they interest you. My experience has been that with time the connections between your interests will make themselves clear."

- "Seek out mentors. Additionally, pursue those mentors who are helpful to you. Make them mentor you."

- "Seek out training that will improve your organizational skills. To survive in this setting, organization is essential. Consider reading David Allen's *Getting Things Done* (New

York: Penguin Books, 2003) and Jim Loeh and Tony Schwartz's *The Power of Full Engagement: Managing Energy, Not Time is the Key to High Performance and Personal Renewal* (New York: Free Press, 2003). I found both of these books to be invaluable."

STORIES FROM THE FRONT LINES: FAVORITE ANTECDOTES OF FACULTY CLINICIANS

This section of the chapter is for enrichment and for fun. It shows what might lie ahead for you, by listening to the voices of current faculty. I asked each of our contributors to tell a favorite anecdote about their experience in academic medicine. I described my request as: "Please tell an anecdote—a story that is meaningful to you—about your experience in academic medicine." The responses are diverse, and not all contributors supplied us with an anecdote. I found it interesting what the individual contributors selected to share in response to an open-ended request. As author of the book, I have made a few editorial comments (in italics). From those contributors who replied, here are the stories:

Role Modeling

"At a national meeting, a colleague approached me and said she really admired one of the presentations in which I had participated. It meant a lot to me that she had noticed, because I hadn't thought much about that particular session. That taught me that senior faculty have to be role models, all the time, because we don't know who will be watching us."

(As an editorial comment, I would add that the advice holds for all faculty—junior and senior—as we are also role models for medical students and residents.)

Writing a Paper and Becoming an Expert

"A few years ago, one of my residents reported a case study of a patient with acetaminophen poisoning. I helped him with the paper and was listed as third author. My involvement in the project was one of helping him organize his findings and write the paper. I did not have any special knowledge of the topic. Over the next few years, I had telephone calls from two attorneys in different parts of the country, inviting me to testify in court as an expert on acetaminophen poisoning. I became aware that publication of even one paper makes you an 'expert,' and you can be tracked down readily on the Web."

(Clinicians aren't the only ones who do MEDLINE searches.)

Mustn't Grumble (Too Much)

"In my first academic position, I was too critical of situations around me that looked like important problems. I was pulled aside and told, 'You cannot help make anything better by calling it ugly.' This was important advice and helped me soften my judgments."

(You never want to become labeled as a "negative" person.)

Sometimes Good Luck Changes Your Career

"When I was completing my fellowship, I was unable to get a job in academic medicine. Therefore I was considering a position in private practice in another city when the following event occurred. I had presented my research data at a national meeting of my specialty and was at a research dinner with faculty from both my fellowship and an academic institution in the city I was moving into. One faculty member leaned over to the other and said, 'Do get this person a position on your faculty.' This actually occurred by cobbling some 'soft money' together, with the agreement that I would obtain NIH funding within several years. For the first year in academia I worked full-time, although paid only a half-time salary. The rest is history."

(Yes, and the "history" is that this faculty member is now a very successful associate dean of a medical school.)

The Role of the Personal Physician

"One day we had a great example of the power of the personal physician. In our primary care clinic, patients are assigned to individual residents, including interns. One day, I was making hospital rounds with our team, including an intern near the end of his first year. As it happened, one of the intern's patients had had acute chest pain overnight and had been admitted to the coronary care unit. We arrived at the patient's bed at the same time as the cardiac surgery team. The nationally renowned chief of the cardiac surgery team patiently explained to the patient why he should have heart surgery and should have the procedure done that morning.

The patient then turned to my intern and asked, 'Doctor, should I have this surgery?'"

Persistence and Leadership

(This story is from another of our contributors who now holds a title of dean.)

"Early in my career, efforts to begin a residency in our hospital fell apart due to political infighting among physicians. The department chair came to work with us to plan what to do next. In his quiet but effective way, the chairman said, 'This is not about this year or next year—it is about the careers of our students and the health of our patients. Persistence and leadership are the best tools to solve this problem.' He was right, and I remember his advice every day."

Does Gray Hair Confer Wisdom?

"Since I entered the academic community much later in life than most, it has been a revelation to me that I am often the senior member in meetings and much to my amazement, people often look to me for advice. This experience 'snuck up on me' and does give me some amusement."

(I, your humble author, also entered academics after years in practice and was flattered when asked for my opinion at

meetings. Because I was only in my forties at the time, it couldn't have been my senior status. I concluded that I had recent, real-life practice experience that most around the academic table lacked.)

Bringing Colleagues Along

(A faculty member who recently moved from one academic medical center to another shares the following story.)

"One of the most enjoyable things I've done is to bring along two members of my research group, both research psychologists. They moved with me last year and I engineered their new appointments as faculty. This is the first faculty position for both of them and they are very much on the early slope of their ascendancy in academic medicine. Our research is highly collaborative and none of us could function well without the others. The concept of pulling others along with me is a richly rewarding one and really one of the main dimensions of this setting."

Giving Back to the Profession

"One observation is the 'town-gown' situation that frequently occurs. Despite the fact that many of the community physicians who practice geographically close to the medical center received either their undergraduate or graduate medical education here, they participate very little in the education of our students and residents. The further I get away from the home institution, the more likely I am to find physicians who are willing to teach medical students (for no direct pay). When you ask them why they do it, they say that it gives them a chance to 'give back to the profession.' I don't fully understand why those who practice nearby do not feel the same. What those who teach discover is that they are energized by the enthusiasm of students who are hungry to develop their clinical skills. I know there are lots of pressures from managed care and so forth. But it's too bad that the 'business' of medicine makes people forget their roots."

The Satisfactions of Teaching

"I find it especially gratifying to train residents in procedural skills. One resident in particular was very interested in learning procedures. When she started working with me, she was frustrated that she could not complete flexible sigmoidoscopies independently; however, she was determined to learn this skill. After a lot of hard work and practice, she left our program skilled and competent in not only flexible sigmoidoscopy but also nasolaryngoscopy and esophagoscopy. There is a lot of professional satisfaction in working with residents to hone their skills so that they can leave your program competent in a particular area."

A Lesson in Interdependence

"Because of my experience as an orthopedic surgeon and a basic scientist who collaborates with veterinarians on pre-clinical research, I was invited as the primary guest lecturer at the Annual College of Veterinary Surgeons meeting, which was an incredible honor and responsibility. It highlighted for me the similarities between the two fields and gave me an understanding of how much interdependence we have in providing evidence-based care to our patients."

The Work Is Hard, but Different

"When I left practice and started a fellowship, I was at a loss for what to do. No interruptions, no phone calls, no calls from patients at home. I sat in the library and read. It was very hard to get used to at first. I think I would have trouble going back to practice again. I'm not sure I could work that hard again. I work hard now, but it's more controlled."

A Note of Thanks

"Recently over the holidays I received a card signed by all the residents at one of the programs where I teach. Each resident had written a short note letting me know how much he or she appreciates my teaching and presence. It was very heartwarming and reinforcing. I do not think that a day goes by that I do not thank my lucky stars for having a job that gives me so much pleasure and fulfillment."

A Risk of Becoming an Academician

(The following anecdote, one of my favorite academic medicine stories, was shared by a friend several years ago. The physician [not one of our listed contributors] had left private practice and, owing to his outstanding organizational skills, had advanced to become an associate dean of a medical school.)

"Not long after I became associate dean, I was home with the family for Thanksgiving dinner. My mother turned to me and inquired earnestly, 'Son, please tell me again what it is that you do now that you aren't a doctor anymore.'"

GENERATIONAL ISSUES

In this chapter about your future and that of academic medicine, I must include a short discussion of the intergenerational tensions that exist among members of the generations of persons found in AMCs. I refer to the Baby Boom generation (born 1945–1962), Generation X (born 1963–1981), and the Millennials (born 1982 and later). You can think of the Baby Boomers as *idealistic*, the Generation Xers as *reactive*, and the Millennials as *civic-minded*. Most medical students, residents, fellows, and young faculty are Generation Xers, maybe even Millennials, whereas senior faculty and administrators are likely to be members of the Baby Boom generation. This would be an insignificant historical footnote if it were not for the noteworthy intergenerational differences in life experiences, personal values, and career expectations of the three groups.

Bickel and Brown have looked at some of these differences and their implications for academic faculty recruitment and development. They describe how "a single generation can come of age in an entirely different milieu than one the previous generation did." Academic senior faculty, largely Boomers, tend to work hard out of loyalty, expect long-term employment, are willing to "pay their dues," believe that self-sacrifice is a virtue, and respect authority. The authors characterize Generation Xers as working hard if balance is allowed, expecting many job searches, believing that "paying dues" is not relevant today, holding that self-sacrifice may have to be endured occasionally, and questioning authority. Dissimilar historical settings help explain the divergence in values and expectations.[1]

Then come the Millennials, aka generation Y, born after 1981. Raines describes the Millennials as focused on children and family; seeking structured lives, keenly aware of terrorism and heroism, and having a multicultural and global perspective. These Millennials, our rising medical students and tomorrow's clinicians, seek creative challenges, believe they are smart and special, are goal-oriented and connected, and are motivated to achieve personally and also serve their communities.[2] Academicians: be advised. These are your future students and residents.

This diversity of belief systems can be seen in the AMC, as students and residents seem to be making important decisions based on anticipated personal lifestyle, while their teachers lament the loss of commitment to services to patients, practice group, and community. As a young faculty member, you will encounter these intergenerational differences daily and must be secure in your own value system and yet seek to understand what others hold dear. Clearly the intergenerational values clash is one of the factors influencing the future of academic medicine.

ABOUT THE FUTURE OF ACADEMIC MEDICINE

The young faculty member should pay attention to the state of academic medicine today. *British Medical Journal* editors Clark and Smith, who wrote an editorial that began, "Academic medicine is in crisis across the world," pointed out the "elephant in the room." "Medicine's capacity to research, think, and teach is collapsing just at a time when science, social trends, and globalization are offering great opportunities—and threats."[3]

What is going on? What is causing the "crisis" in the ability to teach and discover? Clark and Smith cite the imperative to provide clinical service, reduced funding for clinical research programs, and lack of financial incentives, with inadequate rewards for good teachers. A perverse influence is the power of "scientists who bring in large sums from industry."[3] Also, as research has moved from public to private funding, with an emphasis on technology and high-payoff ventures, there has been an attendant subspecialization of research.

Another facet of the academic medicine crisis is the decline in opportunities for academicians to teach, as they struggle to earn their salaries through clinical care and research grants. Richardson writes that once excellent teachers are "at or near extinction, this consequence circles around to become cause, as the absence of such outstanding teaching in the faculty's intellectual DNA means that subsequent generations of learners advance to become teachers without ever having known true excellence in clinical teaching."[4] This image of hereditary educational mediocrity is grim, indeed.

Perhaps the financial stresses of the early 21st century have rekindled the friction between the scholastic and the vocational camps in medicine that has existed since before the days of Flexner.[5] What is really the "greatest good" in the AMC today—clinical income, research funding, or the discovery of new knowledge? Or is it possibly the education of the next generation of America's physicians?

All of this brings me to my hidden agenda for the book: Medical education in the United States began as practitioners shared their often-experiential knowledge and skills with willing apprentices. Following Flexner in 1910, we had "science-based" medical schools—but still with a focus on teaching. The influx of federal dollars that began in the 1960s, and more recently the funding from the pharmaceutical and medical device industries, threaten to convert our treasured academic medical centers into research factories where medical trainees are a disadvantaged minority.

Yet, despite the huge influx of funding, academic medical centers continue to experience financial shortfalls, and they now look to newly hired clinicians for salvation. Perhaps it is providential that the very financial distress that prompts AMCs to hire clinicians to generate practice income might actually resurrect the teaching mission. Although it may not be the plan of the university presidents and hospital administrators, the young clinicians joining faculties are doing so because they want to *teach*. Their presence may just serve to return the academic medical centers to their original mission of training tomorrow's physicians. And, I hope that while in the academic setting, the newly minted academic clinicians also seek intellectual fulfillment through the scholarship of clinical care and teaching.

PLANNING AT YOUR CURRENT CAREER STAGE: WHAT TO DO NOW

From the beginning, I have written this book for four groups of readers: medical students considering an eventual career in academic medicine; residents and fellows who are preparing for academic positions; clinicians practicing in the community who are pondering career changes; and clinician educators in the early stages of their academic lives. At first this might seem like a diverse group, but if you "do the math," you will see that all are likely to be in an age range of about 15 years and be at a time when they must make important life choices.

The following are my career planning suggestions for each group, based on what has been discussed in the previous nine chapters and on the comments of our contributors.

Medical Students Considering Careers in Academic Medicine

If you are a medical student considering an academic career, you are likely to have entered medical school with a little research experience, which you should augment as you move ahead in your career. The important task now is to learn as much as possible about what life is like in the academic world, to accumulate some valuable "tickets" (publications and advanced degrees), and to connect with mentors who can help you achieve your career goals. Here is what I would do, starting today, if I were still a medical student:

- Make your specialty choice as early as reasonably possible. I realize all too well that medical students today are obliged to choose their specialties much too early and based on too little information. However, selecting a specialty path is the key to accomplishing the steps below. If you need some guidance on specialty choice, read Anita Taylor's book *How to Choose a Medical Specialty*[6] or visit the Association of American Medical Colleges (AAMC) Web page on Careers in Medicine.[7]

- Find a career mentor on the faculty, someone who can tell you what academic life is like in your chosen specialty and can help you with residency decisions later. Do this by identifying a faculty member with whom you feel you could communicate well, and then call that person's office and request a 30-minute get-acquainted appointment to discuss your interest in his or her specialty. In almost all instances, the faculty member will be pleased and flattered and will agree to meet with you. At the meetings, ask the questions used in this book, including Why did you choose an academic career? What have been the surprises? What advice do you have for me?

- Find a research mentor, someone who can help you now with a research project, aiming toward publication. This person may or may not be the same as your career mentor.

- Aim for a residency in an academic medical center. In some specialties this is not a significant issue; for example, all neurosurgery residency programs are in AMCs or major referral centers. In other specialties, many—even most—programs are in community hospitals. Community hospital training can give you excellent clinical skills, but to gain the academic success skills you will need (see Chapter 8) and to begin your vital academic networking, you should train in a university-based academic medical center.

- Identify the most respected academic leaders in your field. When you go to national specialty meetings (which you should do as a student interested in an academic career), hunt for these names on the program and attend the sessions they are presenting.

■ Begin even now to think about a career topic (see Chapter 5)—the area of research and speaking that will be your eventual "focus of national expertise."

■ Get to know some senior residents in your intended specialty. By the time you are ready to look for an academic position, these persons may be on faculty and can be helpful in your job search.

Residents and Fellows

Residents and fellows aspiring to academic careers have made the all-important specialty choice and before long may be searching for their first academic position. During your years of specialty or subspecialty training, you should learn some pedagogical skills, continue to accumulate academic "tickets," and extend your network of contacts. I suggest the following:

■ Tell your residency or fellowship director about your academic career aspirations. Then, also speak with your department chair, who probably has nationwide connections that could be helpful to you.

■ Volunteer to do some teaching for medical students or junior residents, in the clinical setting and also in small-group seminars, such as the class in physical diagnosis. This will give you important pedagogical skills and help to build your résumé.

■ Begin a research study, and involve a research mentor from your specialty. Aim for publication in a well-regarded peer-reviewed journal.

■ Prepare a lecture on a clinical topic in your specialty area. Try to find a subject of evolving interest that will continue to be pertinent to clinicians in the future. Then read everything you can on this topic, and keep your Power-Point presentation up to date. Offer to give the lecture to resident and fellow colleagues, and even at continuing medical education programs.

- Go to a national specialty meeting at least once each year. Meet the academic leaders in your field. Volunteer to serve on task forces and committees.
- Begin a file on promising positions in the best academic departments in the country.
- When you are ready to begin your job search during your last year of training, follow the steps described in Chapter 4.

Practicing Community Physicians Considering Academic Careers

Throughout this book, I have stressed the cultural differences between the community practice setting and academia. If you are considering a move from practice to a faculty position, be sure you have read Chapters 1 through 3 very carefully. Then take the following steps:

- Schedule informational appointments with academic leaders in nearby medical schools. These should be clinicians in your specialty, and those who are recognized as successful by their peers. Come to the interviews with questions prepared, based on topics covered in the early chapters of this book. Make your questions open-ended, and don't be afraid to ask the tough questions, such as, "What is likely to be my greatest frustration in academic medicine?" and "What should I do next?" Be sure to ask about whom else you should consult and if you may please call later if you have any questions.
- Think about a clinical focus that might become your career topic. As a full-time practicing physician, you may never be closer to clinical medicine. Your topic will be determined by your specialty and might well be an area that is not already crowded by "experts." For example, there are many experts on hypertension and diabetes mellitus; few are recognized authorities on dizziness or fatigue.
- Prepare and present a lecture on your clinical focus topic. Yes, practicing physicians can do this. Learn to use the PowerPoint program on your computer. Offer to present

your lecture to residents at a nearby training program or to your state specialty society at an annual scientific assembly.

■ If your specialty has an academic society (see Table 8.2), learn about the organization and attend a national meeting.

■ Check with your national specialty academy or academic society to learn about any academic positions open. Contact the institutions offering these positions, and study the job descriptions to find out exactly what is available and the abilities the positions require.

■ Consider applying for an academic position and, if invited, go for the interview. This will be an enlightening experience and, even if offered the job, you can respectfully decline if it does not seem compelling.

■ Think seriously about applying for a faculty development fellowship. This will represent a significant cut in your income for 1 or 2 years, but fellowship training can give you academic skills that will prove vital in your initial job search and in your later academic career. I describe faculty development training in Chapter 9. Keep in mind that fellowships are very diverse and may focus on areas such as teaching, research, health care policy, public health, clinical procedures, or "epispecialties" such as geriatrics, adolescent medicine, or sports medicine.

■ If you decide to make the move, think about the job you want in 10 years, and then plan what you will need to do to qualify for that position.

Faculty Members in Early Career Stages

You have selected your specialty, received necessary residency and fellowship training, and are committed to an academic career—at least for the time being. You realize that you still have a lot to learn about academic medicine.

■ Find a career mentor at your AMC, if you have not already done so.

■ Select a career topic, if you have not already done so. You can always refine or change your choice later, but you cannot allow your scholarly work to remain unfocused too long.

- Prepare a "shelf talk" on your career topic. This is a lecture, generally with a PowerPoint presentation and handout that you keep up to date. If called upon, you should be able to give your "shelf talk" on an hour's notice.

- Get involved in a research project, even if you are not the principal investigator.

- Teach something. This may be a procedural skill workshop for residents, or a seminar for medical students. What's important is honing your teaching skills.

- Join your national academic society, attend the annual meeting, and volunteer for a task force or committee. When you attend national meetings, meet the venerated leaders and the "up-and-coming" young members.

- Present some aspect of your work at a national meeting. This may be part of a joint presentation, which is a good way to learn meeting presentation skills.

- Publish, publish, and publish. Learn early the habit of scholarship and writing.

- Begin planning now for advancement in rank. See Chapter 2 for specific advice on what to do.

- Decide upon the academic position you want next, then collect all the "tickets" you will need to move up.

DOCTOR TAYLOR'S RULES FOR SUCCESS IN ACADEMIC MEDICINE

I will end with some general success strategies that I have always tried to follow.

Seven Rules for Success in Academic Medicine

Throughout this book, I have emphasized the importance of maintaining and perhaps even expanding your clinical skills, becoming involved in scholarly activity, and establishing a mentor relationship. In addition to these fundamental recommendations, I offer the following Rules for Success in Academic Medicine.

Rule 1. Be Willing to Work Very Hard

Academic medicine is no easier or harder than community practice; it is just different. If you enter academics seeking an easier life, you are likely to be disappointed—either by the demanding work required or by the career stagnation that comes if you don't work hard. In July 2005, cyclist Lance Armstrong won the Tour de France race for an unprecedented seventh straight year. When asked the secret of his success, his answer was, "Hard work." He pursued his dream of being the best cyclist in the world. Academic medicine is also a competitive arena and one in which focused effort and endurance can pay off.

Rule 2. Remember to Show Up

In the 1979 movie *Being There*, Peter Sellers plays a mentally challenged gardener who becomes an advisor to the president of the United States by "being there" at critical times, exemplifying the importance of one's physical presence.[8] As a faculty member, there is no substitute for showing up for outpatient clinic, hospital rounds, committee meetings, teaching assignments, and student and resident appointments. It is also important to be present for the nonrequired institutional activities. These include the student white-coat ceremony, university-sponsored social events, hooding and graduation ceremonies, and retirement dinners for colleagues. Who is present and who is not is noticed at special events. Be there.

Rule 3. Take Appropriate Risks

One of our younger contributors tells what she would do differently in her career: "I would not worry so much about taking risks. I would just go for it." It can be hard to believe that, in the staid and venerable halls of academia, the risk-takers come out ahead, but they generally do. Yes, there will be some failures, and that is okay. Not all of your endeavors will succeed and, in fact, if you never, ever fail, you probably aren't taking enough risks. And sometimes, despite careful checking, you will bend a rule. Remember that sometimes it is better to be forgiven than denied.

Sometimes risk taking involves taking the unpopular stand, and at other times you must battle to bring about needed change. The latter can be especially difficult when you are challenging an entrenched system with the motto, "We've always done it that way." When I encounter such a situation, I try to remember that sometimes if you want to be part of the solution, you sometimes have to become part of the problem.

Rule 4. Enjoy Your Work

As a clinician working in an academic medical center, you are one of the most privileged persons on the planet—of all time. You get to work with (sometimes) eager learners, bright colleagues, and patients who need our care. You have unlimited opportunities to expand your intellectual horizons. On a more basic level, you will almost certainly eat well today and sleep in a warm bed tonight. You should give thanks every day for your good fortune, and you should grumble very seldom. Frankly, if you are not enjoying your work immensely, you should probably be doing something else.

Rule 5. Remember Why You Chose to Become an Academic Clinician

Can you recall why you became a physician in the first place? I earnestly hope that it was to help people and, to quote the motto of the Alpha Omega Alpha Honor Medical Society, that you aspire to be "worthy to serve the suffering."[9] As an academic clinician, you have added two more reasons: to teach tomorrow's clinicians and to advance medical knowledge. I urge you to bring passion to your work every day, even if many of the tasks seem mundane.

One of my favorite stories is the parable of the stonecutter. In medieval times, a traveler walking along a road came to a man cutting a stone and asked the stonecutter what he was doing. The reply was, "My job is to make this round rock into a square stone for the mason." This stonecutter did not seem very happy with his job. A little further along the road, the traveler encountered a second stonecutter doing the same job. This workman explained, a little happier than the last, that he was making building blocks that would be used in constructing a church. Even further along the road, the traveler came to a third stonecutter and asked him also what he was doing. This stonecutter smiled with great pride as he replied, "I'm building a cathedral."

The work we do each day is like building a cathedral—of current health services and future practice based on what we teach and discover. Do it joyfully and with pride.

Rule 6. Believe in Yourself

When I was a boy my mother told me over and over, "You can accomplish anything you put your mind to." Your colleagues (or future colleagues) in academic medicine are not super-humans. They are not any smarter than most of the rest of us. They have just followed a specific career path. You can follow a similar path, and do so successfully, if you will just believe in yourself.

Along your career path you will encounter some who will encourage and guide you. You may meet others who can see only failure in your career plans. The experts are sometimes wrong. In 1954, Elvis Presley was fired after one performance at the Grand Ole Opry with the advice: "You ain't goin' nowhere, son. You ought to go back to drivin' a truck."[10] Elvis obviously did not take this advice, and you should likewise be skeptical of those who discourage your highest aspirations. When you make major career decisions, seek advice from those you respect and trust, but in the end you must rely on your own judgment.

You can do it—anything you put your mind to. In the beginning of the book is one of my pet quotations, from a movie based on a story of how Mexican revolutionary Pancho Villa used an American movie company to spread his fame and win U.S. support. The pronouncement is, "The improbability of the events depicted in this film is the surest indication that they actually did occur."

However improbable it might seem, you can actually succeed in academic medicine.

Rule 7. Above All, Maintain Your Personal Integrity

The following comment is by a clinician and friend who has assumed a senior administrative role: "I've found the past five years to be filled with powerful moral choices regarding real conflicts between right and wrong, and the enduring importance of our basic principles and values. As Mark Twain said, 'Always do the right thing. This will gratify some people and astonish everyone else.'"

Always do the right thing, and do it for the right reason. Don't submit a paper for publication because it seems the "right thing" for your career if the paper is second-rate and a waste of the reader's time. Don't join a quality assurance committee unless you really care about quality assurance. Don't choose an academic career if you really don't like teaching and scholarship. As an academic clinician, you must do what is right for all your constituencies: patients, learners, colleagues, your mentors, those you mentor, your family, and for your own conscience.

THE LAST WORDS

My 1978 decision to seek an academic career changed the course of my life, bringing opportunities and experiences I never would have had if I had remained in my comfortable community practice.

I will share a thoughtful quotation from one of our contributors: "My advice is to be true to yourself, pursue your dream, and keep your options open. This advice is for anyone in medicine—whether you are a medical student or an attending-level clinician. It is never too late to make the choice to be happier in life."

After 27 years in academic medicine, I have no doubt that I made the right choice.

REFERENCES

1. Bickel J, Brown AJ. Generation X: implications for faculty recruitment and development in academic health centers. Acad Med 2005;80:205–210.
2. Raines C. Managing millennials. Available at http://www. generationsatwork.com/articles/millenials.htm/.
3. Clark J, Smith R. BMJ Publishing Group to launch an international campaign to promote academic medicine. Br Med J 2003;327:1001–1002.

4. Richardson WS. Letter. JAMA 2004;292:2971.
5. Flexner A. Medical education in the United States and Canada: a report to the Carnegie Foundation for the Advancement of Teaching. New York: Carnegie Foundation, 1910. Available at http://www.carnegiefoundation.org/eLibrary/docs/flexner_report.pdf/.
6. Taylor AD. How to choose a medical specialty, 4th ed. Philadelphia: W.B. Saunders, 2003.
7. Association of American Medical Colleges, Careers in Medicine program. Available at http://www.aamc.org/careersinmedicine/.
8. Based on the novel: Kosinski J. Being there. New York: Harcourt, Brace, Jovanovich, 1971.
9. Alpha Omega Alpha General Information. Available at http://www.alphaomegaalpha.org/AOAmain/General Information.htm/.
10. The problem with experts. Available at http://www.infoPOEMS.com/.

Appendix 1: Glossary

The following terms will be helpful as you read the book. When appropriate, I have listed the chapters where items are chiefly discussed. Fair warning: Some of the terms that follow are fanciful jargon, and I created just a few of them.

ABMS See American Board of Medical Specialties.

Academic clinician A medical practitioner who works in an academic medical center and whose duties include patient care, teaching, and scholarship. See Chapter 1.

Academic health center See Academic medical center.

Academic medical center An institution that combines clinical care, teaching, and scholarship. See Chapter 3.

Accidental plagiarism Unintended plagiarism that occurs when a writer loses track of sources of bibliographic research and subsequently uses another's words as his own, without realizing that he or she is doing so. Using research assistants greatly increases the risk of accidental plagiarism. See Chapter 8.

Adjunct An adjective describing a faculty rank, generally indicating that consideration for promotion cannot be made by the usual standards of the primary faculty. Reasons for adjunct faculty status include serving at an FTE below 0.5, being a full-time employee of another institution, or awaiting review for appointment to a primary faculty rank. See Chapter 2.

Allopathic medicine A system of medicine, chiefly therapeutics, in which a disease is treated by an agent that antagonizes it. The etymologic clue is that the Greek *allos* means "other." Although most have never heard the term, a synonym is "heteropathy," distinguishing allopathy/heteropathy from homeopathy.

Alpha Omega Alpha (AOA)   The medical honor society. Usually one is elected to membership during medical school, but a few residents, faculty, and alumni are inducted each year. See Chapter 3.

American Board of Medical Specialties (ABMS)   An organization consisting of the 24 approved U.S. medical specialty boards. See Chapter 5.

Anticipatory negotiation   The act of preempting a potential opponent's bargaining advantage before a negotiation begins, by making a concession without apparent expectation of gain. See Chapter 7.

BATNA   An acronym for Best Alternative to a Negotiated Agreement. It describes your ultimate fallback position; what you can accept when bargaining breaks down. See Chapter 7.

Burnout   Disabling frustration with one's job, often accompanied by somatic symptoms or manifestations of depression. See Chapter 9.

Career stagnation   Also sometimes called "being stuck." The phrase describes a career state in which there is no progress, no new ideas, flagging energy, and scant hope for advancement. See Chapter 9.

Career topic   The subject that will be the long-term focus of your academic research, speaking and writing, and perhaps your clinical care. See Chapter 5.

Chair; chairman; chairperson; chairwoman   This is the head of a department in a professional school or teaching hospital. With budgetary authority controlling faculty salaries, the chairperson of a department in a school of medicine, nursing, or dentistry can be a very powerful individual. See Chapter 7.

Clinician   One who is qualified to treat sick persons. Clinicians include practicing physicians, nurse-practitioners, and physician assistants.

Compost pile   A pile of papers that might merit responses but probably won't if allowed to "ferment" for a few weeks. This aid to personal time management is discussed in Chapter 7.

Convenience sample   A study cohort selected by an expedient method, such as surveying every patient that came to a single clinic for a week. The book's group of contributors is a convenience sample.

Cos, aka *Kos*   A Greek island that was the home of Hippocrates and the site of an early center of healing, teaching, and scholarship. See Chapter 3.

Curriculum vitae   The written record of your professional accomplishments. In the business world, this is called a résumé, although the format is somewhat different. See Chapter 4.

Data mining   The process of sifting through figures accumulated in a research study, searching for a publishable nugget of data. This is not considered an appropriate research method. See Chapter 6.

Development   A euphemism for fund-raising. See Chapter 3.

Dinosaur   An academician whose knowledge, skills, and organizational abilities have become outdated and who is doomed to extinction—but who may not recognize his or her fate. See Chapter 9.

Direct costs   The NIH Grants Policy Statement defines direct costs as costs that can be specifically identified with a particular project or activity. These typically cover salaries, equipment, supplies, and other specific research project expenses. See Chapter 6.

Doctor   From the Latin word *docere*, meaning to teach. The defining role of the doctor is to educate. One who cares for sick patients is properly called a physician.

Effort allocation   The designation of how one's professional time is divided, typically into categories of clinical practice, teaching, and scholarship. Some governmental effort allocation forms also call for identification of specific funding sources for each professional activity. See Chapter 3.

Epispecialty, aka metaspecialty   A neologism describing an area of special medical expertise that does not represent an official, major medical specialty with board certification. Sometimes epispecialties are formalized with Certificates of Added Qualifications. Examples are geriatrics, sports medicine, and adolescent medicine. See Chapter 3.

Facilities and administrative costs; F&A costs (aka indirect costs)   The NIH Grants Policy Statement defines F&A costs as costs that are incurred by a grantee for common or joint objectives and that, therefore, cannot be identified specifically with a particular project or program. Succinctly stated, F&A costs go to institutional overhead. Also see Direct costs. See Chapter 6.

Faculty track   See Track.

Flexner report   The 1910 document that prompted major reforms in American medical education. See Chapter 3.

Formative evaluation   Also called formative feedback, this report to a learner is intended to change behavior. It is not intended to be a final account of performance (summative evaluation). Formative evaluation may be verbal, written, or both. See Chapter 5.

Fringe benefits (aka other payroll expenses)   What you receive, other than salary, in return for your work. Fringe benefits may include vacation allotment, sick time, health insurance, disability insurance, life insurance, retirement benefits, and more. See Chapter 4.

FTE   See Full-time equivalent.

Full-time equivalent (FTE)   The fraction of a full-time position held by an individual. Thus a full-time job is 1.0 FTE, and a quarter-time job is 0.25 FTE. See Chapter 2.

Generalizability   A bit of scientific jargon that refers to the gold standard for results of a clinical study; that is, that the results of a study can be extrapolated to a larger population. See Chapter 6.

Grantsmanship   The ability to write grants that are approved and funded. Grantsmanship is a highly valued skill in academia. See Chapter 6.

Grasshopper   An academician who submits an abstract to a scientific meeting, with no intention of attending the meeting. His or her only objective is to have the work published in the abstract book for the meeting, so that it can be added to a curriculum vitae. See Chapter 9.

Hard money   Funds that a department and its faculty can usually count on from year to year. This generally refers to the department's base budget from the school, which may in turn come largely from a state allocation. Income from endowments may also contribute to hard money. Also see Soft money. See Chapter 3.

The Health Insurance Portability and Accountability Act of 1996   See HIPAA.

HIPAA, aka HIPPA   The acronym is pronounced sounding like hippopotamus. The Health Insurance Portability and Accountability Act of 1996 was a well-meaning law intended to protect Americans with preexisting medical conditions or who might suffer discrimination in health coverage based on a factor relating to an individual's health. Subsequent regulations interpreting the law have immensely complicated health care in America, and HIPAA is now considered a poster child for the law of unintended consequences. See Chapter 6.

Homeopathic medicine　The Greek word *homoios* means "like, resembling." Homeopathy is based on treating a disease with drugs that can produce symptoms like those of the disease to be treated, the drug being given in very small doses.

Hypothesis　A research theory to be tested by a study, generally presented as a statement. Alternatively, a study hypothesis is sometimes stated as a research question. See Chapter 6.

Impostor syndrome　The feeling that one "really does not deserve to be here." Clinicians with this syndrome live in fear that someone will discover the extent of their incompetence. The impostor syndrome is common among junior faculty in academics; some senior faculty also suffer this disorder. See Chapter 8.

Indirect costs　See Facilities and administrative costs.

Institutional review board (IRB)　An official committee of an academic institution, charged with approving research protocols before the study can commence. The IRB will examine a proposal for patient safety, informed consent, appropriate treatment of animals, and potential ethical concerns. See Chapter 6.

IMRAD　An acronym representing introduction, method, results, and discussion—the major headings in a research report. See Chapter 6.

IRB　See Institutional review board.

Job sharing　Two persons are hired to fill one position, generally with a total of 1.0 FTE. See Chapter 2.

Junior faculty Faculty members holding the ranks of instructor and assistant professor. See Chapters 2 and 3.

Kos See Cos.

Letter of intent A synopsis of a grant concept sent to a grantor as a preliminary step in the application process. If the grantor agrees that the idea may have merit, a full grant proposal may follow. See Chapter 6.

Maintenance of certification (MOC) An evolving process advocated by the American Board of Medical Specialties intended to provide an assessment of a physician's clinical performance that will lead to enhanced practice quality. See Chapter 5.

Mission-based budgeting An attempt to link hard money allocations awarded to academic departments to specific institutional missions, notably education. See Chapter 3.

MOC See Maintenance of certification.

National Institutes of Health (NIH) The NIH describes itself as the steward of medical and behavioral research for the nation. It is an agency of the U.S. Department of Health and Human Services and receives more than $28 billion yearly in Congressional appropriations.

NIH See National Institutes of Health.

NIH shunt A career advancement shortcut in which someone leaving a position at the National Institutes of Health lands a coveted position in an academic medical center for which some might say he or she gained advantage by virtue of NIH experience. See Chapter 8.

NOGA See Notice of grant award. Used as an acronym, NOGA is pronounced rhyming with toga. Receiving a NOGA is a good thing, sometimes followed by a celebration. See Chapter 6.

Notice of grant award (NOGA)   The official statement that you have received a grant for your project, telling how much money you are eligible to receive over what length of time. See Chapter 6.

One-minute-preceptor   A widely used structured method of clinical teaching. See Chapter 5.

Osteopathic medicine   Osteopathy is a system of therapy that emphasizes the value of normal structural relationships, proper nutrition, and a favorable environment. Its practitioners use generally accepted medical and surgical methods, with a focus on attaining normal body mechanics, often through manipulation.

Other payroll expenses (OPE)   See Fringe benefits.

Physician   One who is qualified to practice medicine.

Precepting; preceptor   Teaching in the clinical setting in relation to a specific patient. See Chapter 5.

Program officer (aka project officer)   An agent of a granting agency who has administrative responsibility for a specific grant project. The program officer can be a big help as you prepare a grant. See Chapter 6.

Project officer   See Program officer.

Proposal concept paper   See Letter of intent.

Provider   A derogatory term, coined by government and third-party payers, to describe those who "provide" medical care. A preferred term is clinician, or more specifically physician.

Qualitative research   Research that is more concerned with descriptive content than with numerical data. Qualitative research is typically used when the research question is behavioral or social, complex in nature, and inappropriate for quantitative methods. See Chapter 6.

Quantitative research Research that involves collecting numerical data. Quantitative research involves testable hypotheses, measurable variables, and inferences drawn from samples that can be extrapolated to a larger population. See Chapter 6.

Reciprocity norm A social belief system that holds that if I perform a favor or service, I can expect one in return— even if not from the person who received the original favor. See Chapter 7.

Recreational data collection The process of accumulating research data just because it can be done, with very little likelihood that it will ever be used. See Chapter 6.

RFP See Request for proposal.

Reproducibility Based on what is included in a report of clinical research, a knowledgeable investigator could conduct the same study—although the results may or may not mirror those in the original report. See Chapter 6.

Request for proposal An invitation by a funding agency to submit a grant proposal. There will be dollar limits, a deadline, and—very important—a statement of the type of proposals most likely to be approved. See Chapter 6.

Research question See Hypothesis.

Restrictive covenant An agreement that prohibits a physician from leaving a medical group and beginning a subsequent, competing practice in a specified geographic location. See Chapter 4.

Scholarly imperative A term describing the importance of scholarship to faculty. Scholarly work may take many forms. See Chapter 3.

Scud missile An angry memo, now generally launched by e-mail, aimed at an individual or small group. See Chapter 8.

Senior faculty Faculty members holding the ranks of associate professor and professor. See Chapters 2 and 3.

Shadow charts Duplicate patient care records that faculty clinicians maintain in their academic offices. These will probably become of historical interest when electronic medical records become fully functional and readily available on all academic medical center computers. See Chapter 5.

Shelf talk A lecture, generally on your career topic, that you keep up to date and could "take off the shelf" and present within an hour's notice. See Chapter 10.

Significance; significant In statistics, a significant finding is one that very likely did not occur by chance. Statistical significance is a measurement of the probability that the finding might be the result of chance, commonly less than 5%. See Chapter 6.

Soft money Money that the department cannot count on from year to year. This generally refers to grant funding, although there are other sources of soft money. Also see Hard money. See Chapter 3.

Stuck See Career stagnation.

Summative evaluation A formal evaluation of an individual's performance. In an educational setting, a report card is a summative report. Also see Formative evaluation. See Chapter 5.

Target journal When writing a scientific paper, the target journal is your first-choice site for publication. See Chapter 6.

TBA An abbreviation for "to be added." As an example, TBA might refer to a faculty member to be hired if a grant proposal is funded. See Chapter 6.

Tenure   An academic status that has some implications, but not necessarily a guarantee, regarding job security. See Chapter 2.

Terminal rank   Signifies that one's current rank is as far as one will advance in his or her career. See Chapter 3.

Testosterone storm   A whimsical term for a gender-specific malady in which a male faculty member develops a compelling obsession with a woman (not his wife) and cannot resist the urge to engage in self-destructive behavior. See Chapter 8.

Ticket   In the academic sense, a "ticket" is something that helps qualify you for a position or opportunity. A ticket may be tangible (a degree after your name or a publication), experience (such as being able to perform a very specialized procedure), or useful knowledge (such as how to get an NIH grant). See Chapter 10.

Tournament funding competition   A tongue-in-cheek description of how we joust for grant support. See Chapter 6.

Track   A term describing a faculty appointment. Various types of faculty tracks are described in Chapter 2.

Triple-threat academician   A clinical faculty member who sees patients, teaches medical students or residents, and conducts (and publishes) research. The term is borrowed from football, where it describes a player who can run, pass, and kick. Some say that both the triple-threat academician and gridiron star are becoming anachronisms. See Chapter 1.

Up-or-out policy   An institutional rule that requires a faculty member to be promoted at the end of a specific time, often 7 years, or risk termination of employment. See Chapter 2.

Upward delegation When savvy staff members or junior faculty members succeed in having a chore that is really their job performed by someone holding superior rank. See Chapter 9.

War stories Anecdotal tales of past clinical exploits or woes, beloved by senior faculty and endured by learners. See Chapter 5.

WIRMS An acronym for "What I Really Mean to Say." Using this exercise can help a writer get started or "unstuck" on a paper. See Chapter 6.

X, Y, and Z A system that describes the sources of an academic salary in which X represents base salary, Y indicates payment for pedagogical or administrative duties, and Z is practice-generated income. See Chapter 2.

Appendix 2: Collected Academic Medical Aphorisms

Medical aphorisms are the physician's secret indulgence. We physicians relish the aphorism—the succinctly stated truth. I can still remember the exact times in medical school when I first heard, "When you hear hoof beats, don't look for zebras," and "All that wheezes is not asthma."

Medical academia, with a long heritage of bright people working in often challenging situations, offers an especially rich treasury of aphorisms. I have collected many of the aphorisms scattered through this book and listed them here. Wise physicians and educators created most of these aphorisms, and I have cited authors when I could find the sources. The original authors of many are lost in the mists of history, although their words have become part of the lore of medicine. I created a few of the sayings that follow.

Here they are, sorted by chapter:

About This Book
- If you have seen one academic medical center, you have seen one academic medical center.
1. Deciding on an Academic Career
- We who love academic medicine are always seeking to clone ourselves.
- In academic medicine, being a good clinician is not enough.
2. About an Academic Career
- The third year of medical school marks the transition from the precynical to the cynical years.
- Your tenure is your clinical skills.
- In the medical school, students are an underrepresented minority.
3. What You Need to Know About the Academic Medical Center

- Creating new knowledge is what academic medical centers do best.

4. Finding the Academic Job You Want
   - Your record gets you the interview; your interview gets you the job.
   - Academic job recruitment is like courtship; we are on our best behavior, but the end may not be a long-term relationship.
   - Make your deals on the doorstep.
   - A university is a loose federation of departments united by a common parking problem. (Recently, a colleague in Florida stated that, in that state, what links departments is air-conditioning ducts.)

5. Basic Academic Skills: Clinical Practice, Teaching, and Scholarship
   - "The three priorities in teaching are first, to inspire; second, to challenge; and third and only third, to impart information." (J. Michael Bishop)
   - "To teach is to learn twice." (Joseph Joubert)
   - Academic medicine adores reductionism.

6. Advanced Academic Skills: Doing Research, Getting Grants, and Writing for Publication
   - Learn the skill of delegating without abdicating.
   - Good writing can't fix bad research.
   - Research is a team sport; writing (at least, composition) is a solo activity.
   - Do not let the perfect become the enemy of the good.
   - With patience and perseverance, there is a journal home for the well designed, carefully conducted, clearly reported study.

7. Administrative Skills
   - Do your own work first.
   - Sometimes meetings actually get work done.
   - Influence is having your views represented when a decision is made; power is being at the table for the decision.
   - Where meetings are held matters.
   - Never go into a decision-making meeting without knowing exactly what you want from the meeting.

- "When you are talking, you aren't learning anything." (Lyndon Johnson)
- Any discussion can last much longer than anticipated.
- No project is so logical, beneficial, and safe that your institution's legal department can't kill it. (Modified from *Dilbert*)
- Leaders build castles in the sky, and managers charge rent on those castles.
- Power used is power lost.
- You can change the world if only you don't care who gets credit.
- "If you fail to plan, you are planning to fail." (Benjamin Franklin)

8. Academic Medicine Success Skills
   - Don't be smart in school and dumb on the bus.
   - We fight so hard because the stakes are so low.
   - He who goes to the law holds a wolf by the tail.

9. How to Manage Your Career and Your Life
   - Turn your work into play, and then play hard.

10. Planning for the Future
    - Academic medicine is no easier than community practice; it is just different.
    - It is sometimes better to be forgiven than denied.
    - Sometimes if you want to be part of the solution, you need to become part of the problem.
    - If you aren't enjoying your career immensely, you should probably be doing something else.
    - Always do the right thing, and do it for the right reasons.

Appendix 3: Allopathic Medical Schools in the United States

The following lists accredited United States MD-granting medical schools. The Web site for full information is http://www.aamc.org/medicalschools.htm.

Alabama
University of Alabama School of Medicine
Birmingham, AL 35294-3293

University of South Alabama College of Medicine
Mobile, AL 36688

Arizona
University of Arizona College of Medicine
Tucson, AZ 85724-5018

Arkansas
University of Arkansas College of Medicine
Little Rock, AR 72205

California
Keck School of Medicine of the University of Southern California
Los Angeles, CA 90033

Loma Linda University School of Medicine
Loma Linda, CA 92350

Stanford University School of Medicine
Stanford, CA 94305-5119

University of California, Davis, School of Medicine
Davis CA 95697-8640

University of California, Irvine, College of Medicine
Irvine, CA 92697-3950

David Geffen School of Medicine, UCLA
Los Angeles, CA 90095

University of California, San Diego, School of Medicine
La Jolla, CA 92093

University of California, San Francisco, School of Medicine
San Francisco, CA 94143-0410

Colorado
University of Colorado Health Sciences Center School of
Medicine
Denver, CO 80262

Connecticut
University of Connecticut School of Medicine
Farmington, CT 06030

Yale University School of Medicine
New Haven, CT 06520-8055

District of Columbia
George Washington University School of Medicine and
Health Sciences
Washington, DC 20037

Georgetown University School of Medicine
Washington, DC 20007

Howard University College of Medicine
Washington, DC 20059

Florida
Florida State University College of Medicine
Tallahassee, FL 32306-4300

University of Florida College of Medicine
Gainesville, FL 32610

University of Miami School of Medicine
Miami, FL 33101

University of South Florida College of Medicine
Tampa, FL 33612-4799

Georgia
Emory University School of Medicine
Atlanta, GA 30322

Medical College of Georgia School of Medicine
Augusta, GA 30912

Mercer University School of Medicine
Macon, GA 31207

Morehouse School of Medicine
Atlanta, GA 30310

Hawaii
University of Hawaii John A. Burns School of Medicine
Honolulu, HI 96822

Illinois
Rosalind Franklin University of Medicine and Science/The
Chicago Medical School
North Chicago, IL 60064

Loyola University Chicago Stritch School of Medicine
Maywood, IL 60153

Northwestern University Medical School
Chicago, IL 60611-3008

Rush Medical College of Rush University
Chicago, IL 60612

Southern Illinois University School of Medicine
Springfield, IL 62794-9620

University of Chicago Division of the Biological Sciences Pritzker School of Medicine
Chicago, IL 60637-1470

University of Illinois College of Medicine
Chicago, IL 60612

Indiana
Indiana University School of Medicine
Indianapolis, IN 46202-5114

Iowa
University of Iowa Roy J. and Lucille A. Carver College of Medicine
Iowa City, IA 52242-1101

Kansas
University of Kansas School of Medicine
Kansas City, KS 66160-7300

Kentucky
University of Kentucky College of Medicine
Lexington, KY 40536-0298

University of Louisville School of Medicine
Louisville, KY 40202-3866

Louisiana
Louisiana State University School of Medicine in New Orleans
New Orleans, LA 70112-2822

Louisiana State University School of Medicine in Shreveport
Shreveport, LA 71130-3932

Tulane University School of Medicine
New Orleans, LA 70112

Maryland
Johns Hopkins University School of Medicine
Baltimore, MD 21205

Uniformed Services University of the Health Sciences/F. Edward Hebert School of Medicine
Bethesda, MD 20814-4799

University of Maryland School of Medicine
Baltimore, MD 21201

Massachusetts
Boston University School of Medicine
Boston, MA 02118

Harvard Medical School
Boston, MA 02115

Tufts University School of Medicine
Boston, MA 02111

University of Massachusetts Medical School
Worcester, MA 01655-0112

Michigan
Michigan State University College of Human Medicine
East Lansing, MI 48824

University of Michigan Medical School
Ann Arbor, MI 48109-0624

Wayne State University School of Medicine
Detroit, MI 48201

Minnesota
Mayo Medical School
Rochester, MN 55905

University of Minnesota Medical School–Twin Cities
Minneapolis, MN 55455

Mississippi
University of Mississippi School of Medicine
Jackson, MS 39216

Missouri
Saint Louis University School of Medicine
St. Louis, MO 63104

University of Missouri-Columbia School of Medicine
Columbia, MO 65212

University of Missouri-Kansas City School of Medicine
Kansas City, MO 64108-2792

Washington University in St. Louis School of Medicine
St. Louis, MO 63110

Nebraska
Creighton University School of Medicine
Omaha, NE 68178

University of Nebraska College of Medicine
Omaha, NE 68198-6545

Nevada
University of Nevada School of Medicine
Reno, NV 89557-0046

New Hampshire
Dartmouth Medical School
Hanover, NH 03755-3833

New Jersey
UMDNJ–New Jersey Medical School
Newark, NJ 07103-2714

UMDNJ–Robert Wood Johnson Medical School
Piscataway, NJ 08854-5635

New Mexico
University of New Mexico School of Medicine
Albuquerque, NM 87131

New York
Albany Medical College
Albany, NY 12208

Albert Einstein College of Medicine of Yeshiva University
Bronx, NY 10461

Columbia University College of Physicians and Surgeons
New York, NY 10032

Joan & Sanford I. Weill Medical College of Cornell University
New York, NY 10021

Mount Sinai School of Medicine of New York University
New York, NY 10029-6574

New York Medical College
Valhalla, NY 10595

New York University School of Medicine
New York, NY 10016

State University of New York Downstate Medical Center College of Medicine
Brooklyn, NY 11203-2098

State University of New York Upstate Medical University
Syracuse, NY 13210

Stony Brook University Health Sciences Center School of Medicine
Stony Brook, NY 11794-8430

University at Buffalo State University of New York School of Medicine & Biomedical Sciences
Buffalo, NY 14214

University of Rochester School of Medicine and Dentistry
Rochester, NY 14642

North Carolina
Duke University School of Medicine
Durham, NC 27710

The Brody School of Medicine at East Carolina University
Greenville, NC 27858-4354

University of North Carolina at Chapel Hill School of
Medicine
Chapel Hill, NC 27599

Wake Forest University School of Medicine
Winston-Salem, NC 27157

North Dakota
University of North Dakota School of Medicine and Health
Sciences
Grand Forks, ND 58202-9037

Ohio
Case Western Reserve University School of Medicine
Cleveland, OH 44106-4915

Medical College of Ohio
Toledo, OH 43699-0008

Northeastern Ohio Universities College of Medicine
Rootstown, OH 44272-0095

Ohio State University College of Medicine and Public Health
Columbus, OH 43210-1238

University of Cincinnati College of Medicine
Cincinnati, OH 45267-0555

Wright State University School of Medicine
Dayton, OH 45401-0927

Oklahoma
University of Oklahoma College of Medicine
Oklahoma City, OK 73190

Oregon
Oregon Health & Science University School of Medicine
Portland, OR 97239-3098

Pennsylvania
Jefferson Medical College of Thomas Jefferson University
Philadelphia, PA 19107-5083

Drexel University College of Medicine
Philadelphia, PA 19129

Pennsylvania State University College of Medicine
Hershey, PA 17033

Temple University School of Medicine
Philadelphia, PA 19104-6055

University of Pennsylvania School of Medicine
Philadelphia, PA 19104-6055

University of Pittsburgh School of Medicine
Pittsburgh, PA 15261

Puerto Rico
Ponce School of Medicine
Ponce, PR 00732

Universidad Central del Caribe School of Medicine
Bayamon, PR 00960-6032

University of Puerto Rico School of Medicine
San Juan, PR 00936-5067

Rhode Island
Brown Medical School
Providence, RI 02912

South Carolina
Medical University of South Carolina College of Medicine
Charleston, SC 29425

University of South Carolina School of Medicine
Columbia, SC 29208

South Dakota
University of South Dakota School of Medicine
Sioux Falls, SD 57105-1570

Tennessee
East Tennessee State University James H. Quillen College of
Medicine
Johnson City, TN 37614

Meharry Medical College School of Medicine
Nashville, TN 37208

University of Tennessee Health Science Center College of
Medicine
Memphis, TN 38163

Vanderbilt University School of Medicine
Nashville, TN 37232

Texas
Baylor College of Medicine
Houston, TX 77030

Texas Tech University Health Sciences Center School of
Medicine
Lubbock, TX 79430

The Texas A & M University System Health Science Center
College of Medicine
College Station, TX 77843-1114

University of Texas Medical School at San Antonio
San Antonio, TX 78229-3900

University of Texas Southwestern Medical Center at Dallas
Southwestern Medical School
Dallas, TX 75390

University of Texas Medical Branch at Galveston
Galveston, TX 77555

University of Texas Medical School at Houston
Houston, TX 77030

Utah
University of Utah School of Medicine
Salt Lake City, UT 84132-2101

Vermont
The University of Vermont College of Medicine
Burlington, VT 05405

Virginia
Eastern Virginia Medical School
Norfolk, VA 23501

University of Virginia School of Medicine Health System
Charlottesville, VA 22908

Virginia Commonwealth University School of Medicine
Richmond, VA 23298-0565

Washington
University of Washington School of Medicine
Seattle, WA 98195-6340

West Virginia
Joan C. Edwards School of Medicine at Marshall University
Huntington, WV 25701-3655

West Virginia University School of Medicine
Morgantown, WV 26506

Wisconsin
Medical College of Wisconsin
Milwaukee, WI 532226

University of Wisconsin Medical School
Madison, WI 53706

Appendix 4: Osteopathic Medical Colleges in the United States

The following lists United States DO-granting medical schools. The Web site for full contact information is http://www.aacom.org/colleges.

Arizona
Arizona College of Osteopathic Medicine of Midwestern University
Glendale, AZ 85308

California
Touro University College of Osteopathic Medicine
Vallejo, CA 94592

Western University of Health Sciences/College of Osteopathic Medicine of the Pacific
Pomona, CA 91766-1854

Florida
Nova Southeastern University College of Osteopathic Medicine
Ft. Lauderdale, FL 33314-7796

Illinois
Chicago College of Osteopathic Medicine of Midwestern University
Downer's Grove, IL 60515

Iowa
Des Moines University College of Osteopathic Medicine
Des Moines, IA 50312

Kentucky
Pikeville College School of Osteopathic Medicine
Pikesville, KY 41501

Maine
University of New England College of Osteopathic Medicine
Biddeford, ME 04005

Michigan
Michigan State University College of Osteopathic Medicine
East Lansing, MI 48824

Missouri
Kansas City University of Medicine and Biosciences College
of Osteopathic Medicine
Kansas City, MO 64106-1453

Kirksville College of Osteopathic Medicine
Kirksville, MO 63501

New Jersey
University of Medicine and Dentistry of New Jersey School
of Osteopathic Medicine
Stratford, NJ 08084

New York
New York College of Osteopathic Medicine of The New York
Institute of Technology
Old Westbury, NY 11568-8000

Ohio
Ohio University College of Osteopathic Medicine
Athens, OH 45701-2979

Oklahoma
Oklahoma State University Center for Health Sciences/
College of Osteopathic Medicine
Tulsa, OK 74107

Pennsylvania
Lake Erie College of Osteopathic Medicine
Erie, PA 16509

Philadelphia College of Osteopathic Medicine
Philadelphia, PA 19131

Texas
University of North Texas Health Science Center at Fort Worth/Texas College of Osteopathic Medicine
Fort Worth, TX 76107-2699

Virginia
Edward Via Virginia College of Osteopathic Medicine
Blacksburg, VA 24060

West Virginia
West Virginia School of Osteopathic Medicine
Lewisburg, WV 24901

Appendix 5: Medical Schools in Canada

The following lists accredited Canadian MD-granting medical schools. The Web site for full information is http://www.aamc.org/members/listings/msgeocanada.htm.

Alberta
University of Alberta Faculty of Medicine and Dentistry
Edmonton, AB
Canada T6G 2R7

University of Calgary Faculty of Medicine
Calgary, AB
Canada T2N 4N1

British Columbia
University of British Columbia Faculty of Medicine
Vancouver, BC
Canada V6T 1Z3

Manitoba
University of Manitoba Faculty of Medicine
Winnipeg, MB
Canada R3E 0W3

Newfoundland
Memorial University of Newfoundland Faculty of Medicine
St. John's, NF
Canada A1B 3V6

Nova Scotia
Dalhousie University Faculty of Medicine
Halifax, NS
Canada B3H 4H7

Ontario
McMaster University School of Medicine
Hamilton, ON
Canada L8N 3Z5

Queen's University Faculty of Health Sciences
Kingston, ON
Canada K7L 3N6

The University of Western Ontario Faculty of Medicine &
Dentistry
London, ON
Canada N6A 5C1

University of Ottawa Faculty of Medicine
Ottawa, ON
Canada KIH 8M5

University of Toronto Faculty of Medicine
Toronto, ON
Canada M5S 1A8

Quebec
Laval University Faculty of Medicine
Quebec City, PQ
Canada G1K 7P4

McGill University Faculty of Medicine
Montreal, PQ
Canada H3G 1Y6

Universite de Montreal Faculty of Medicine
Montreal, PQ
Canada H3C 3J7

Universite de Sherbrooke Faculty of Medicine
Sherbrooke, PQ
Canada J1H 5N4

Saskatchewan
University of Saskatchewan College of Medicine
Saskatoon, SK
Canada S7N 5E5